Checklist

Esscll

~

Medical Checklists

Series Editors: Alexander Sturm
Felix Largiadèr
Otto Wicki

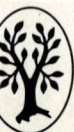

Georg Thieme Verlag Stuttgart · New York
Thieme Medical Publishers, Inc., New York

Checklist
Intensive Care Medicine

Including Poisoning

Hans-Peter Schuster, Tiberius Pop,
Ludwig Sacha Weilemann

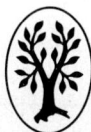

1990
Georg Thieme Verlag Stuttgart · New York
Thieme Medical Publishers, Inc., New York

Library of Congress Cataloging-in-Publication Data

Schuster, Hans-Peter.
[Checkliste Intensivmedizin. English]
Checklist intensive care medicine : including poisoning /
Hans-Peter Schuster, Tiberius Pop, Ludwig Sacha Weilemann.
(Medical checklists)
Translation of: Checkliste Intensivmedizin.
Includes bibliographical references.
1. Critical care medicine--Handbooks, manuals, etc. I. Pop. T.
II. Weilemann, Ludwig Sacha, III. Title. IV. Series.
[DNLM: 1. Critical Care--handbooks. 2. Poisoning--handbooks. WX
39 S395c] RC86.8.S3813 1989

Important Note: Medicine is an ever-changing science. Research and clinical experience are continually broadening our knowledge, in particular our knowledge of proper treatment and drug therapy. Insofar as this book mentions any dosage or application, readers may rest assured that the authors, editors and publishers have made every effort to ensure that such references are strictly in accordance with **the state of knowledge at the time of production of the book. Nevertheless, every user is requested** to carefully examine the manufacturer's leaflets accompanying each drug to check on his own responsibility whether the dosage schedules recommended therein or the contraindications stated by the manufacturers differ from the statements made in the present book. Such examination is particularly important with drugs which are either rarely used or have been newly released on the market.

1st German edition 1983   1st Turkish edition 1988
2nd German edition 1985   3rd German edition 1988

Cover design by D. Loenicker, Stuttgart

This book is an authorized and revised translation of the third German edition, published and copyrighted 1988 by Georg Thieme Verlag, Stuttgart, Germany. Title of the German edition: Checkliste Intensivmedizin, einschließlich Vergiftungen.

© 1990 Georg Thieme Verlag, Rüdigerstrasse 14, D-7000 Stuttgart 30, Germany
Thieme Medical Publishers, Inc., 381 Park Avenue South, New York, N. Y. 10016
Typesetting and printed by Druckhaus Götz KG, D-7140 Ludwigsburg
(System 5 [202] Linotype). Printed in West-Germany

ISBN 3-13-724901-5 (Georg Thieme Verlag, Stuttgart)
ISBN 0-86577-320-3 (Thieme Medical Publishers, Inc., New York)   1 2 3 4 5 6

To
Renate, Marlies, and Irene

Authors' and Series Editors' Addresses

Prof. Felix Largiadèr, M.D., M.S. (Minn.)
Chairman, Department of Surgery and Director,
Visceral Surgery Division
University Hospital
8091 Zürich
Switzerland

Prof. Tiberius Pop, M.D.
IInd Department of Medicine Hospital
Johannes Gutenberg University
Langenbeckstrasse 1
6500 Mainz
Federal Republic of Germany

Prof. Hans-Peter Schuster, M.D.
Ist Department of Medicine Hospital
City Hospital and Teaching Hospital of the Hannover Medical School
Weinberg 1
3200 Hildesheim
Federal Republic of Germany

Prof. Alexander Sturm, M.D.
Director, Department of Medicine Hospital
Ruhr University Bochum
Marienhospital
4690 Herne/Westphalia
Federal Republic of Germany

Prof. Ludwig S. Weilemann, M.D.
IInd Department of Medicine Hospital
Johannes Gutenberg University
Langenbeckstrasse 1
6500 Mainz
Federal Republic of Germany

Otto Wicki, M.D.
6707 Iragna
Switzerland

Series Editors' Preface to the Medical Checklists

The Checklists of state-of-the-art medicine are intended as sources of information and for quick reference. Their handy dimensions permit them to be kept within reach, granting the physician rapid orientation on:

– the most relevant leading and secondary symptoms of a disorder;
– essential and important diagnostic examinations;
– conservative and (in appropriate cases) surgical therapeutic options;
– differential diagnostic and differential therapeutic considerations in problematic and important disorders.

The Checklists are no substitute for diagnostic compendiums or comprehensive textbooks, nor are they intended as such; essentially, they are logically arranged mnemonic aids. To maintain a concise structure without oversimplifying the content, most of the points have been formulated as incomplete sentences. Orderly presentation of up-to-date information on diagnosis and treatment has intentionally been given priority over scientific references and descriptions of very rare disease entities.

The Checklists were designed to meet the needs of practicing physicians not specialized in the individual disciplines, as well as those of practitioners from all fields, and advanced students. The Checklists contain three sections:

– The first section, identified by gray page headings, is concerned with techniques of examination in and away from the hospital.
– The second section, identified by blue page headings, is concerned with etiology, pathogenesis and clinical symptomatology, findings and procedures relevant to diagnosis, differential diagnostic considerations where appropriate, and conservative treatment of specific disorders.
– The third section, identified by red page headings, contains brief descriptions (i.e., as much as necessary for each specialty) of potential indications for surgery, principle and technique of the operation, and/or suggestions for intensive care and management.

To date, the following Checklists have been published in German:

– Conservative medicine: "Vascular System – Hypertension", "Endocrinology and Metabolism", "Intensive Medicine", "Oncology", "Gastroenterology", "Hematology", "Cardiology", "Pneumology", "Dermatology and Venerology", "Imaging Methods", "Psychiatry and Neurologic Emergencies"
– Surgical disciplines: "Urology", "Visceral Surgery", "Gynecology", "Orthopedics", "Traumatology", "Pediatric Surgery", "Ambulant Surgery", and "Application of Casts"

In addition, a Checklist on "Nursing Care" has appeared.

This Checklist of Intensive Care Medicine is the first to be published in the English language. We wish it the same success that it has received in the original language.

We are deeply indebted to Georg Thieme Publishers, especially to Drs. G. Hauff and D. Bremkamp for their energetic support and realization of this concept, which has been a cooperative endeavor.

Herne-Bochum, Zürich, Iragna

Alexander Sturm
Felix Largiadèr
Otto Wicki

Authors' Preface

This book was written for everyone engaged in intensive medicine. We are thoroughly aware of the risk undertaken in presenting a Checklist of Intensive Care Medicine for publication. More than in other fields, treatment of intensive care patients requires comprehension of pathophysiology and adaptation of therapy to the individual situation. Worldwide clinical and basic research on pathophysiology, pathobiochemistry, and therapy of the critically ill has resulted in rapid publication of a glut of data as a foundation for therapeutic notions, some of which change swiftly. Nevertheless, we have accepted the challenge, out of a conviction that intensive medicine has reached the stage at which generally valid criteria for admittance to the intensive care unit and intensive management and treatment can be identified and verbalized.

This has provided the basis for dividing the book into three sections: Intensive care unit monitoring; management of typical disorders encountered in intensive care units, including poisonings and standard methods of parenteral alimentation; and infusion therapy (input-output balancing, mechanical ventilation, cardiopulmonary resuscitation, electrotherapy, pharmacotherapy, and extracorporeal waste elimination procedures). All major sections have been assembled and subdivided in similar fashion to aid the reader in locating desired information.

We hope that we have succeeded in depicting both basics and generally accepted standards of intensive care medicine without too frequently overstepping the limits imposed by schematic structures. The authors have also taken the liberty of expressing personal views on a few topics!

Mainz, October 1989   The Authors

Abbreviations

$A\text{-}aDO_2$	Alveolar-arterial O_2 partial pressure
ABG	Arterial blood gas
ACE	Angiotensin converting enzyme
ACTH	Adrenocorticoid hormone
ADH	Antidiuretic hormone
AIDS	Acquired immune deficiency syndrome
AP	Alkaline phosphatase
APACHE	Acute physiology and chronic health
ARDS	Adult respiratory distress syndrome
ARF	Acute renal failure
ASB	Assisted spontaneous breathing
ASV	Assisted spontaneous ventilation
AT III	Antithrombin III
ATP	Adenosine triphosphate
AV	Atrioventricular
aVF	Augmented volt, foot (ECG)
aVR	Augmented volt, right arm
A wave	Atrial wave
BAL	British anti-lewisite
BP	Blood pressure
bpm	Beats per minute
BUN	Blood urea nitrogen
BW	Body weight
C	Compliance
CAPD	Continuous ambulatory peritoneal dialysis
CAT, CT	Computerized Axial Tomography, -gram; computed tomography
CBC	Complete blood count
CCU	Critical care unit
CK	Creatine kinase
CK-MB	Creatine kinase, cardiospecific
cm	Centimeter
CNS	Central nervous system
C.O.	Cardiac output
CPD	Continuous peritoneal dialysis
CPAP	Continuous positive airway (end-expiratory) pressure
CPK	Creatine phosphokinase
CPK-MB	Cardiospecific CPK
CPPV	Continuous positive-pressure ventilation
CSF	Cerebrospinal fluid
CVP	Central venous pressure
DIC	Disseminated intravascular coagulation
DPG	Diphosphoglyceric acid
D/W	Dextrose in water
ECG	Electrocardiography, -gram
ECMO	Extracorporeal membrane oxygenation
EDH	Euhydration, dehydration, hyperhydration
EEG	Electroencephalography, -gram
EIP	End-inspiratory pressure
ELISA	Enzyme-linked immunosorbent assay

ENT	Ear, nose, throat
Fr	French (Charrière)
FRC	Functional residual capacity
FSP	Fibrinogen split products
GI	Gastrointestinal
GOT	Glutamate-oxalate transferase
GPT	Glutamate-pyruvate transferase
Hb	Hemoglobin
Hct	Hematocrit
HIG	Hyperimmune globulin
HIV	Human immune deficiency virus
HR	Heart rate
HTLV-3	Human T-cell leukemia virus, type 3
IABA	Intraaortic balloon assist
i-aDO$_2$	Inspiratory-arterial O$_2$ partial pressure
ICU	Intensive care unit
IgA	Immoglobulin A
IgG	Immoglobulin G
IM	Intramuscular
INH	Isonicotinic acid hydrazide
IPD	Intermittent peritoneal dialysis
IPPB	Intermittent positive-pressure breathing
IPPV	Intermittent positive-pressure ventilation
IU	International unit
IV	Intravenous
LDH	Lactate dehydrogenase
L-T$_3$	Liothyronine
MCV	Mean corpuscular volume
Met	Methionine
MI	Mitral insufficiency or myocardial infarction
MMV	Mandatory minute ventilation
MOV	Minimal occlusion volume
MV	Minute volume
PA	Pulmonary arterial
PEEP	Positive end-expiratory pressure
PEG	Percutaneous endoscopic gastroscopy
PNPV	Positive-negative pressure ventilation
PTT	Prothrombin time
PVR	Pulmonary vascular resistence
PWA	Pulmonary wedge arterial
RBC	Red blood cell/count
SA	Sino-atrial
SCPPV	Synchronized continuous positive-pressure ventilation
SGG	Standard gamma globulin
SGOT	Serum glutamic-oxaloacetic transaminase
SIMV	Synchronized intermittent mandatory ventilation
SLE	Systemic lupus erythrematosus
SMMV	Synchronized mandatory minute ventilation
STH	Somatotropic hormone

Abbreviations

THAM	Tris-hydroxylmethyl aminomethane (tris)
TISS	Therapeutic intervention scoring system
TSH	Thyroid-stimulating hormone
TT	Thrombin time
U_{Osm}	Urine osmolality
U/P	Urine/plasma osmotic ratio
WBC	White blood cell/count
WPW	Wolf-Parkinson-White syndrome
ZAP	Zero airway pressure

Contents

Contents

Contents

Principles – Indications – Techniques

- Besides electronic and laboratory data monitoring, direct physical examination and observation of the intensive care patient by the attending physicians and nursing personnel is of central importance in the ICU (intensive care unit) setting, as elsewhere. It requires both methodical, scheduled examinations and emergency workups that may be prompted by specific data or situations. No patient may be exempted from this practice.

Inspection:
- Patient's overall condition
- Signs of agitation or pain
- Seizures
- Turgor
- Condition of skin and mucous membranes
- Cutaneous circulation and/or lesions
- Respiratory movements
- Girths
- Positioning and joint alignment
- Position, orifice of entry, and security of attachment of catheters, drains, and tubes

Auscultation:
- Appropriate position of respiratory and gastrointestinal tubes
- Pulmonary ventilation
- Bronchial secretions
- Pulmonary infiltrations
- Heart sounds and murmurs
- Intestinal sounds

Palpation:
- Tenderness
- Turgor
- Catheterized blood vessels
- Precordial movements
- Abdominal muscle tone

Percussion:
- Accumulation of fluids
- Thoracic ventilation
- Meteorism and flatulence

Neurology:
- Level of consciousness
- Response when spoken to
- Reflexes
- Pupils
- Response to painful stimuli

Documentation and Execution of Procedures

- All ICU monitoring must be carried out in accordance with a previously established time schedule at defined intervals. This applies both to written orders for the nursing personnel and to examinations done by physicians.
  - A basic framework is provided by routine morning and evening rounds and one check of specific problems during the night. The course must be documented in writing both in the morning and in the evening.
  - Beyond this, constant, direct contact with the patient must be maintained. Every conspicuous change must be reported to the attending physician, who therefore must always be available and present in the ICU.
- All data on examinations done and observations made by the nursing staff must be entered with the proper time in the supervision protocols.

Principle

- Electronic monitoring refers to continuous surveillance of biologic functions by means of electronic instruments. The objects of measurement are bioelectric signals; the derivation system runs from a sensor or receiver on the patient via lead cables and impulse amplifiers or converters to TV (television) monitors that provide continuous display of the functions undergoing evaluation (Fig. 1).

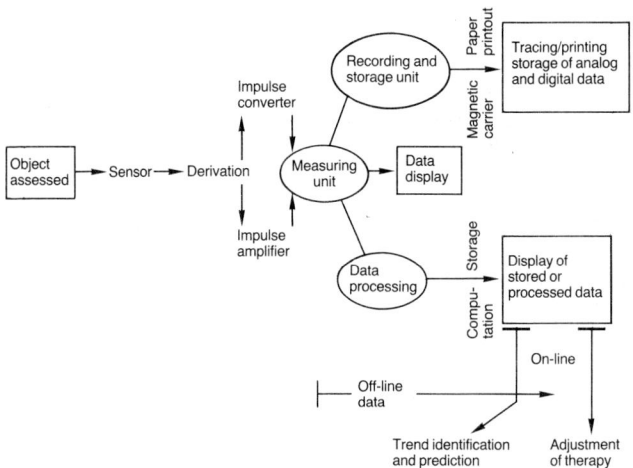

Fig. 1   Diagram of electronic patient-monitoring setup

- Requirements for electronic monitoring systems are as follows:
  - Continuous recording of the functions being monitored = continuous display
  - Immediate detection of critical deviations of the biologic functions being measured = critical-value alarm
  - Early identification of potentially dangerous deviations of the biologic parameter being measured = trend alarm (still largely experimental)
- The most advanced automatic data storage and retrieval systems utilize computer-supported data processing systems. On- and off-line data are stored in a computer memory, processed by a program, and the requested results displayed on a monitor screen or printed out, as desired. Computer-supported surveillance systems

Table 1   Means of bedside monitoring

Objects measured	Method	Recorded and derived parameters
Circulatory system		
Cardiac action potentials	Skin electrodes	ECG, heart rate, extrasystoles
Pulse waves	Optical transmission sensors, pressure sensors	Pulse tracings, pulse rate, Δ heart-pulse rate
Blood pressure	Intraarterial cannula/ catheter, Statham element, catheter-borne micromanometer	Force of pulsation, systolic and diastolic blood pressures, mean blood pressure
CNS		
Brain waves	External adhesive electrodes or intracutaneous needle electrodes	EEG
Intracranial pressure	Intracranial pressure sensors	Intracranial pressure
Body temperature		
Rectal temperature	Thermistor probe	Temperature tracing,
Skin temperature	Thermistor loop	Δ rectal/skin temp.
Respiratory system		
Breathing mechanics	Thermistor probes/ spirometry, thoracic cage impedance	Tracing of respiratory cycle, respiratory rate, duration of apnea
Respiratory volumes	Spirometry	Inspiratory volume, minute volume
Airways pressure	Pressure sensors, membrane manometer, potentiometer	End-inspiratory, end-expiratory, and mean airway pressures; compliance, resistance
Blood gases		
intravascular	Catheter-borne electrodes, polarography	pO_2
	Catheter-borne electrode, Severinghaus' principle	pCO_2
	Diffusion-membrane catheter, mass spectrometry	pO_2, pCO_2
	Fiberglass optical catheter, reflection oxymetry	O_2 saturation

Table **1** (continued)

Objects measured	Method	Recorded and derived parameters
transcutaneous	Heated skin electrodes, polarography	pO_2
	Earclip oxymetry	O_2 saturation
Composition of exhaled air	Exhaled air sample, mass spectrometry	pO_{2E}, pCO_{2E}, FO_{2E}, FCO_{2E} O_2 consumption, energy turnover
Metabolism		
Acid-base status, blood sugar	Continuous aspiration of blood, external flow electrode, autoanalyzer (hexose-kinase method)	pH, pCO_2, $[HCO_3^-]$, glucose concentration

of greatest importance are those for detection of arrhythmias and for monitoring measurement data and computed parameters of cardiocirculatory function and fluid balance.

Indications

- Many biologic functions are accessible to electronic monitoring (Table **1**)), although there are considerable differences in practicability and clinical experience.
- The basic monitoring program must include ECG (electrocardiogram) and heart rate surveillance. For patients with acute cardiovascular disorders (acute myocardial infarction, heart surgery) continuous monitoring of intravascular pressures has become standard procedure.
- The selection of other functional parameters for monitoring depends on the type of patient and the equipment available. It is not possible to make universally valid recommendations.
- Continuous EEG (electroencephalogram) monitoring is probably done too rarely. It is indicated in cases of acute poisoning or metabolic coma, following cardiopulmonary resuscitation, during status epilepticus and in relaxed patients undergoing mechanical ventilation.

- Monitoring systems built into therapeutic instruments (dialysis monitors, ventilator monitors, monitors in infusion and injection pumps) have attained widespread practical significance. They serve to control the function of the instruments themselves, and the electronic equipment of modern respirators also permits surveillance of other biologic events. Monitoring of total thoracic compliance during controlled ventilation and of energy turnover based on indirect calorimetry via measurement of O_2 consumption and rate of CO_2 elimination in the ventilated patient (recently developed "metabolic computers") are important examples.

Instruments – Technique

Monitoring equipment

- Data on monitored parameters may be displayed as functional curves on an oscilloscope (analog signals), clockface dials, or as numerical data (digital signals).

- The ECG monitor should be equipped with a short-term electronic memory capable of storing information for a few seconds prior to an event of interest, and from which the information can be retrieved.

- The monitoring device should be equipped with a critical-value optical and acoustical alarm that is set off by deviation from previously defined limits of the parameter concerned.

- The monitoring device should be connected to a recording unit. As a rule, curves (analog signals) are traced by paper scribers that may be turned on selectively, and can record emergency events when automatically switched on by the critical-value alarm. The short-term data immediately preceding such events must be included in the recording as well.

- Numerical (digital) data may be printed out at selected intervals. They may also be displayed on a TV screen as curves based on discrete data recorded over a protracted period, or as dotted tracings on paper (trend display or trend scriber).

- In combination with electronic storage and calculating systems (computer-supported monitoring), stored data may be displayed in the form of tables or curves showing the course of a functional parameter versus time. To date, this elaborate version of electronic surveillance is available only in a few specialized hospitals; final appraisal of its usefulness in treatment of critically ill patients is not yet possible.

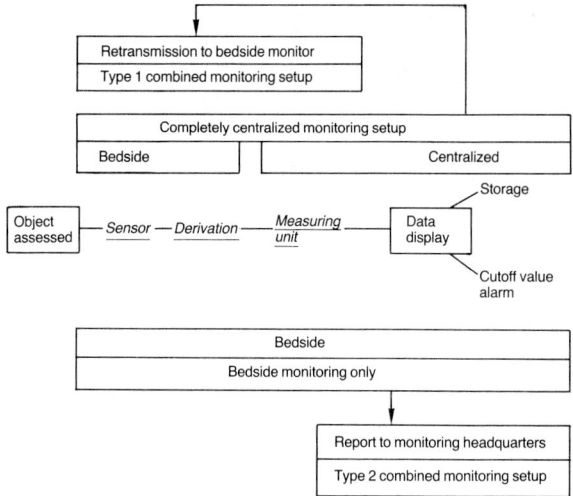

Fig. 2   Basic arrangements for supervision of monitoring

Monitoring Systems (Fig. **2**)

- Centralized surveillance system: Information is passed on via a preamplifier to a central unit, where it is displayed on a TV screen.
  Advantage: data on vital functions of several patients observable from one spot
  Drawback: lack of direct bedside information
- Bedside surveillance system: All operations (derivation, processing, and display of data) are performed by a bedside monitor.
  Advantage: availability of complete information at each patient's bed
  Drawback: lack of overview of data at a central point in the unit
- Combined surveillance system Type I: Data are compiled by a central system and are referred back to a bedside daughter monitor.
  Drawback: complete dependence of the daughter monitor on the central system
- Combined surveillance system Type 2: Data derived and processed by bedside monitors are returned to the central system, where they are displayed in combination.
  Advantage: independence of the bedside monitors from the central unit
  Drawbacks: larger dimensions of the bedside units; high cost

Nursing Aspects

- The potential contribution to the efficiency of the nursing staff ("electronic nurse") has been largely overrated.

  Although monitoring of simple parameters, e.g., heart rate, respiration rate, and body temperature, has relieved the attendants of a few bedside tasks, modern monitoring techniques, e.g., continuous intravascular assessment of blood pressure or blood gases, require additional work. The primary justification of electronic monitoring is that it provides optimum surveillance of the patient as a foundation for better treatment and management, and not that it improves the efficiency of routine care.

Principle

- Indwelling IV (intravenous) catheter with its tip in the major intrathoracic venous system, which lacks valves; appropriate position is in the superior vena cava, but position in one of the brachiocephalic veins is tolerable
- Access route both for measurement of central venous pressure and for continuous IV infusions

Indications

- Measurement of central venous pressure (see p. 28).
- Administration of long-term IV drips in:
  - Balanced infusion therapy (see p. 208).
  - Parenteral nutrition (see p. 202).
  - Elimination of poisons by forced diuresis (see p. 199).
- Continuous or frequent administration of medication

Techniques

- Central venous catheters ("lines") are introduced via percutaneous venipuncture. Typical points of access are:
  - Cubital vein (cubital cannulation)
  - Subclavian vein (subclavian cannulation)
  - Internal jugular vein (jugular cannulation)
- Advantages and drawbacks of cubital vein cannulation:
  - Easily and rapidly performed, uncomplicated venipuncture
  - Frequent inappropriate placement of the catheter tip, which may enter the contralateral jugular or subclavian vein
  - High incidence of thrombotic complications
  - Interference with arm mobility
- Advantages and drawbacks of subclavian cannulation:
  - Rapid venipuncture, feasible even in case of shock or cardiocirculatory arrest
  - Little interference with bodily movement
  - Some hazard of life-threatening complications of puncture (pneumothorax, hematothorax, infusion thorax)
- Advantages and drawbacks of jugular cannulation:
  - Low incidence of complications
  - Complicated venipuncture technique
  - Danger of infection in the presence of a tracheostomy

Central Venous Catheter

- Selection of access route depends on physician's experience and practice, available time, and the patient's overall situation. Subclavian puncture should be avoided:
  - During positive-pressure ventilation, especially positive end-expiratory pressure
  - In case of bleeding tendency
  - During thrombolytic treatment
- *Equipment:*
  IV catheter, tourniquet, disinfectant solution, local anesthetic, sterile drape, sterile gloves, fluid-filled (isotonic saline) hypodermic syringe, venous pressure gauge
- *Sites of venipuncture:*
  - Basilic vein: elbow crease
  - External jugular vein: following compression of the vessel above the clavicle, about in the middle of the sternocleidomastoideus muscle
  - Internal jugular vein: below the angle formed by the external jugular and the sternocleidomastoid at the level of the superior thyroid notch. The trocar must be held at a 45°, vertical angle and the needle advanced toward the clavicular insertion of the muscle
  - Subclavian vein (infraclavicular approach): midclavicular insertion of the trocar, advancement toward the upper border of the sternoclavicular joint
  - Subclavian vein (supraclavicular approach): between lateral border of sternocleidomastoid muscle and clavicle; advancement of trocar at an angle of 45° to the sagittal plane and 15° to the horizontal plane

Complications

- A distinction must be made between complications incurred
  a) while introducing the catheter:
  - Trauma
  - Catheter embolism
  - Inappropriate position
  b) once the catheter is in situ:
  - Thrombophebitis
  - Infection, sepsis
  - Catheter embolism
- Traumatic complications
  1. Inadvertent puncture of the adjacent artery or injury to the vein can lead to extensive hematoma, or, in case of subclavian cannulation, to hematothorax. Arteriovenous fistulas may develop following trauma to an artery.

2. Trauma to pleura or lungs (especially in case of subclavian catheters) may result in life-threatening pneumothorax, tension pneumothorax, or subcutaneous emphysema.
3. Advancement through the adventitia or perforation of a venous wall may result in infusion or transfusion thorax.

- Embolic obstruction of the catheter, i.e., embolism by avulsed catheter fragments, may result from improper technique, either by damage to the catheter by the puncturing needle on introduction, or from inadequate care and surveillance of a long-residing catheter.
  Embolized catheter fragments must be removed either by special transvenous procedures or by thoracotomy.

- The most frequent complication at introduction of venous catheters is inappropriate placement.
  1. The most dangerous position is when the tip of the catheter comes to rest in the right atrium or right ventricle, where it may give rise to arrhythmias or fatal mural perforation with cardiac tamponade.
  2. Remember:
     The position of the catheter is affected by movements of the head and body. The catheter tip may move up to 7 cm caudal when head and trunk are flexed forward. This must be considered in evaluating roentgenograms; the tip of the catheter should lie several cm proximal to the right atrium.
  3. Some typical malpositions:
     - Catheter tip in the axillary vein or the subclavian vein
     - Cranial deviation of the catheter with advancement into the internal jugular vein
     - Contralateral deviation of the catheter with advancement into the subclavian, axillary, or jugular vein of the opposite side
     - Lateral deviation of a subclavian catheter into the axillary vein
     - Looping of the catheter
  4. All deviations of the catheter tip into a smaller vein (axillary, subclavian, external jugular veins) involve an increased hazard of thrombosis; moreover, the pressure readings in the axillary or external jugular vein do not reflect central venous pressure.
     Loop formation increases the risk of phlebitis and pressure necrosis.

Central Venous Catheter

- The most frequent complication of long-residing IV catheters is local venous thrombosis.
  1. The incidence of catheter-induced thrombosis is inversely related to the venous diameter at the point of insertion, and directly related to the length of the segment occupied by the catheter. Thus thrombophebitis is less common in subclavian catheters, and far less so in internal jugular catheters than in cubital vein catheters.
  2. Figures reported on incidence of thrombosis in clinical studies (total 4–10%, cubital cannulation 8–10%, subclavian cannulation 0.5%, internal jugular cannulation 2%) are probably too low.
     The incidence of thrombosis increases with duration of catheter use.
     a) Acute inflammatory thrombophlebitis of the catheter-bearing vein is painful, but heals well once the catheter is removed.
        Treatment:
        – Elevation of the arm
        – Local cooling, ointment dressings with salves containing antiinflammatory agents and heparin
        – Systemic administration of antiinflammatory agents in appropriate cases
        – Anticoagulation
     b) Insidious development of thrombophlebitis may not be noticed until signs of congestion occur after removal of the catheter; resolution of such infections is poor.
        Treatment:
        – Evaluation of indications for vascular surgery or thrombolysis
        – Anticoagulation
        – Compression dressing
  3. In case of doubt, phlebography of the affected arm is indicated.
- The most dangerous complication of long-residing catheters is sepsis emanating from infection of the catheter.
  1. Incidence of catheter sepsis is reported to range from 1–7%, the average being 2–3%. Colonization of the tip of the catheter with pathogens occurs much more frequently (20–40%). The incidence of sepsis increases with the time the indwelling catheter is in situ.
  2. Not every sepsis of obscure origin in a patient with an indwelling catheter is necessarily due to the catheter. Association does not imply a causal relationship. Still, in all patients with venous catheters and an unknown septic focus, the catheter must be considered a potential source. In case of doubt the venous line should be removed, if compatible with surveillance of vital functions. Otherwise, a blood culture must be obtained and antibiotic treatment initiated immediately thereafter, in accor-

dance with the general rules for initial treatment of sepsis (see p. 245).

3. Proof of catheter sepsis consists of resolution of fever following removal of the venous catheter, and demonstration of the septic pathogens in the tip of the catheter.

Prevention of Complications: Care of the Catheter

- Stringent indication criteria for central venous cannulation
- Appropriate handling of venipuncture equipment in accordance with the manufacturer's instructions
- Aseptic precautions upon introduction of the catheter
- Roentgenographic verification of the position of the catheter, if necessary after filling the catheter with contrast medium (see p. 47):
  - Roentgenographic verification immediately following insertion of the catheter
  - Correction of position if necessary, and documentation of the new position
  - Repeated subsequent checks of position, since the catheter may slip
- Fixation of the catheter at its point of emergence by special adhesive dressing
- Daily change of dressing:
  - Check for edema, redness, visible egress of fluid at puncture site
  - Cleansing of the skin around the puncture site with disinfectant sprays or solutions
- Removal of the catheter in case of phlebitis, thrombosis, suspected infection, if compatible with the patient's vital situation
- Strict hygienic precautions when connecting and changing infusions, injecting drugs into the IV catheter or the lines leading to it, and when measuring central venous pressure
- Continuous administration of heparin considerably lessens the risk of thrombosis. In patients not already on anticoagulants for other reasons, heparin may be added to the other drips in a dosage appropriate for prevention (see p. 302).

Principle – Indications – Equipment

- A urinary bladder catheter serves
  - to assess urinary output;
  - to prevent complications of urinary incontinence;
  - to provide access for irrigation in the event of bleeding.
- Every unconscious or semiconscious patient requires a urinary bladder catheter, but so do conscious patients with problems of fluid balance.
- *Two routes of access* are available:
  1. Transurethral catheterization
     Advantage: technical simplicity
     Drawback: higher risk of infection and mucosal trauma
  2. Suprapubic bladder puncture
     Advantage: lower risk of infection, no mucosal trauma to the urethra
     Drawback: more difficult insertion technique
- In any case, sterile precautions are necessary to maintain a closed bladder drainage system as long as the catheter is in situ. Every disconnection between catheter and receptacle multiplies the risk of infection many times over.

Documentation

- Measurement and documentation of urinary output is the responsibility of nursing personnel on written orders by a physician. The following procedure serves well:
  1. Routine readings at 4-h intervals
  2. Hourly readings in the event of oliguria
  3. Measurement of amount of urine accrued in each 12-h period (let urine run off via special valve), with assessment of osmolality (specific gravity) and dipstick tests for glucose, acetone, and blood
  4. 24-h collection for computation of creatinine clearance and for other, optional examinations pertaining to specific problems (e.g., electrolytes, phosphate, toxic substances)

Complications

- Occlusion
  Remember:
  Whenever diuretics are to be given for anuria, patency of the catheter must first be confirmed by inspection!
- Local and ascending infections
- Mucosal damage
- Hemorrhage
- Following bladder drainage, careful observation of the patient is warranted, as voiding difficulties due to functional and/or pathologic-anatomic defects may occur.
  Remember:
  So-called bladder training by clamping off the catheter is nonsensical and conducive to ascending infection.

Gastrointestinal Intubation

Principle – Indications

- An indwelling plastic tube is introduced through the inferior nasal meatus and advanced to the stomach. It is useful in diagnosis, treatment, control of fluid balance, and general surveillance. It is indispensible in unconscious and semiconscious patients, as well as in intubated patients.
  1. In diagnosis:
     - pH assessment of gastric secretions
     - Toxicologic analysis of gastric secretions
     - Early recognition of hemorrhage
     - Recognition of copremesis in the event of intestinal obstruction
  2. In treatment:
     - Neutralization of gastric secretions
     - Feeding
     - Irrigation in the event of bleeding
  3. Monitoring of fluid homeostasis:
     - Measurement of amount of gastric secretion, and analysis for electrolyte loss if appropriate
     - Prevention of aspiration of gastric juices
     - Monitoring in case of bleeding
- Special indications:
  1. Gastric tube suction for aspiration in case of stomach atony, pyloric stenosis, pancreatitis, intestinal obstruction, or peritonitis
  2. Small-intestinal tube for enteric administration of nutrients
  3. Double-barreled tube with gastric and enteric openings (see p. 250).

Technique

Depending on the indication, a polyurethane or silicon rubber tube with a single or double lumen. Vinyl is not suitable because of the softeners it contains. Smallest gauge for diagnostic purposes: 15 Fr.

- Plastic single-lumen tube (special situations may require a double lumen) at least 14 Fr in diameter in best. The tubes should be cooled prior to use.
  - A cold tube is easier to advance.
  - A lubricant should be used.
  - Spray to prevent sticking should be applied to the tube before insertion.
  - The tube is inserted through the inferior nasal meatus and passed through the inferior concha, then

Gastrointestinal Intubation

- advanced into the esophagus, which is facilitated by inclining the head forward until it touches the chest.
- If difficulties arise, a Magill forceps may be used to advance the tube under visual control.
- Correct position must be verified by auscultation.

- Continuous aspiration can be achieved by siphoning (use a graduated receptacle with a capacity of at least 1000 mL, containing 500 mL water) or a suction pump.
- A small-intestinal tube may be placed under visual control by endoscopy, or advanced by natural peristaltic action, and the position verified by x-ray.

Documentation

- Measured volumes of gastric secretion must be documented in writing. Intervals for determining fluid balance must be established in advance and should be at least 12 hours long.
- If more than 500 mL gastric fluid is lost in 24 hours, or another related problem arises, electrolyte loss via gastric fluid must be considered in the input-output balance (see p. 129).

Complications

- Mucosal trauma
- Perforation of the esophagus
- Excessive advancement, so that the tube comes to lie in the small intestine
- Kinking of the tube
- Apposition to the stomach wall
- Trauma to gastric mucosa by tube that is too stiff

Nursing Aspects

- Correct fixation of the nasogastric tube to the external nasal meatus prevents pressure ulceration and mucosal injury due to excessive mobility of the tube.
- Ensure patency.
- Check position daily.

Principle

- Drains ensure egress of accumulated fluid and air from normal anatomic or pathologic body cavities and crevices.
- Of greatest significance in the ICU are:
  - Peritoneal drains
  - Pleural drains
  - Mediastinal drains
  - Pericardial drains

Indications

- Peritoneal drainage:
  - Treatment of peritonitis
  - Removal of toxic substances from the abdominal cavity in the presence of free tryptic enzymes there
  - Drainage of accumulated fluid from the abdominal cavity
  - Drainage of abscesses
  - Irrigation via surgically placed drains (e.g., in acute purulent peritonitis or necrotizing pancreatitis)

  Remember:
  Indication and region to be drained must be documented in writing by the surgeon.
- Pleural drainage permits:
  1. Release of trapped air in pneumothorax, regardless of source
  2. Drainage of abnormal fluid accumulations in inflammatory and noninflammatory conditions
     - Drainage is via closed vacuum system.
- Mediastinal and pericardial drainage: to permit release of abnormal fluid accumulation of inflammatory or noninflammatory origin, or following surgery

Instruments – Techniques

Always use disposable drains.
- Peritoneal drainage
  - Sterile precautions are required for insertion of drainage tubes not placed during surgery. A trocar with drainage catheter or a disposable introduction set may be used; the latter is less dangerous, and sterility is better.
  - Every drainage tube must be carefully secured. Wound edges must be meticulously approximated.

- Pleural drainage
  - In the event of iatrogenic pneumothorax (by subclavian catheter or positive pressure ventilation), emergency drainage of the pleural cavity should be carried out by a physican well versed in intensive medicine.
  - New chest x-rays are required before invasive treatment is initiated, except in life-threatening emergencies due to tension pneumothorax.
  - The drainage catheter is inserted via trocar after stab incision, preferably with a sterile disposable set.
  - Sterile conditions must be established and precautions carefully observed.
  - Incision and insertion are as a rule in the 4th or 5th intercostal space in the posterior axillary line, which is the proper position to drain fluid, but not air. The instrument pierces the skin in the sagittal plane until it touches a rib, is then aimed tangentially upward through the next higher intercostal space and into the pleural cavity. The catheter is advanced to the level of the 1st or 2nd intercostal space.

    Alternative route:

    Incision and insertion in the 2nd intercostal space in the mid-clavicular line

  Remember:

  For fluid drainage, select the lowest point of the pleural cavity in the posterior axillary line or midscapular line (usually at the level of the 8th or 9th rib).

  - Vacuum pump should be connected immediately; check for effectiveness and adjust suction accordingly.
  - Examine the wound for tight closure and proper fixation of the drain.
  - Chest x-ray must be taken for verification and documentation of correct position; sonographic assessment in appropriate cases.
- *Pericardial drainage:* see Pericardial Tamponade, p. 81.

Documentation

- Amounts of fluid drained must be measured and documented. Times for which fluid input-output balance is to be computed must be established in advance (intervals of no less than 12 hours).
- When several drains are present, each corresponding region must be documented and considered separately in the balance.
- Suction strength must be checked and documented at regular intervals.

Complications

- Peritoneal drainage:
  - Bleeding, vascular trauma
  - Intestinal trauma
  - Blockage of flow
  - Infection – Entry of pathogens
  - Loss of protein and electrolytes
- Pleural drainage:
  - Trauma to intercostal vessels
  - Trauma to the lung
  - Infection – Entry of pathogens
  - Compromise of ventilation and circulation due to elevated pressure when drain is obstructed
  - Invasion of a bronchus (must be considered when the effect of otherwise adequate suction is too small)

Nursing Aspects

- An understanding of the region drained by each catheter and the indication for drainage is essential for intelligent, thorough control and care of drains.
  This implies appropriate briefing and alertness for possible complications.
- Fluid balance data must be carefully recorded.
- Dressings must be changed and drains examined for proper function at regular intervals established by written order.

Principle

- Clinical and electronic monitoring must be supplemented by analysis of certain chemical, hematologic, and clotting parameters at regular intervals.
- A distinction must be made between a basic battery of laboratory tests appropriate for all ICU patients and optional specialized testing protocols. The basic battery of tests must be accessible at all times of day or night, whereas it is usually sufficient to perform specialized or follow-up testing at usual times in a routine laboratory.

Indications

- The basic protocol is required for all critically ill patients on admission to the ICU and at least once in the 24-h period thereafter.
  An abbreviated version of the basic protocol is justified for patients in cardiac ICUs.
  - Basic protocol: See Table **2**.
  - The basic protocol must include analysis of blood gases and acid-base status, blood counts, electrolytes, blood glucose, BUN (blood urea nitrogen), total protein, hepatic enzymes, global clotting tests, and urinalysis.
  - Serum lactic acid assessment is highly desirable. Hyperlactatemia is common in ICU patients, and the lactic acid level is of predictive value at least in circulatory shock, cardiocirculatory arrest, and acute poisoning. It is useful in assessment of severity and course of all critical illness states. Increasing or consistently high lactic acid concentrations are always indicative of an unfavorable course or complications that require a change in therapeutic regimen.
  - Osmolalities of serum and urine are highly desirable. They are of great value in identification and management of disorders of fluid and electrolyte balance, as well as for early recognition of acute renal failure, and are also useful as overall predictors.
  - Assessment of oncotic pressure of plasma and edema fluid has not yet become established practice. The weighting it should receive in ICU practice is still controversial. Plasma oncotic pressure aids in differentiating pulmonary edema of cardiac origin from that due to permeability disorders, and may be of predictive significance.
  - Awareness of activities of hepatic enzymes, CK (creatine kinase) CK-MB (cardiospecific CK), and lipase in serum is necessary for confirmation and course evaluation in emergency diagnosis of myocardial infarction, hepatic disease, pancreatitis, and exogenous poisoning.

21

Table 2   Basic laboratory analysis protocol for intensive care patients

---

Blood gases and acid-base status

Serum levels
- Glucose
- Total protein
- Creatinine, urea (BUN)
- Sodium, potassium
- [Lactic acid]

Serum activities
- SGOT
- [CK (CK-MB)]
- [Lipase]

Hematology
- Hemoglobin
- RBC count
- WBC count
- Hematocrit

Clotting parameters
- Platelet count
- PTT
- Quick's test
- Thrombin time
- Fibrinogen level
- [Fibrin(ogen) split products]
- [Reptilase time]
- [Antithrombin III]

Urinalysis
- Glucose
- Protein
- Acetone

[Toxicology tests]
- Blood alcohol
- Cholinesterase activity
- Co-Hb
- Met-Hb

[CSF tests]
- Cell count
- Cell types
- Total protein
- Glucose

[ ] = only in special cases; see text

- In ICUs in which cases of poisoning are treated, assays for cholinesterase activity, CO (carbon monoxide), methemoglobin, and blood alcohol levels should be available.
- Intensive care of neurologic and neurosurgical patients requires examination of cerebrospinal fluid for cell count, cell types, glucose levels, and total protein content.
- Assessment and treatment of convulsions requires assays of phenobarbital and phenytoin levels.
- Evaluation of intravascular clotting disorders and hyperfibrinolysis, which are common in ICU patients, depends upon global coagulation tests (PTT [prothrombin time], Quick's test, thrombin time, platelet count), assay of fibrinogen level, fibrin(ogen) split products, reptilase time, and antithrombin III activity. Assessment of plasminogen levels (which decrease during enhanced fibrinolysis) and prekallikrein in plasma (which drops when intravascular clotting is enhanced) is desirable.

Technics – Organization

- Basic testing can be carried out either in a small laboratory within the ICU or in a special emergency service of a centralized laboratory. The routine department of a centralized laboratory should not be expected to provide appropriate around-the-clock service.
- Advantages and drawbacks of a laboratory within the ICU:
  - Immediate analysis of specimens without delays (particularly blood gases and lactic acid)
  - No transportation problems
  - Direct communication of findings and immediate personal contact in case questions arise
  - Availability of bedside assay units for blood gas analysis, blood sugar, lactic acid, clotting tests, osmometry, and oncometry

  Drawbacks:
  - Costly 24-h availability of a laboratory technician *or*
  - Loss of time for care and treatment (if tests must be done at odd times by ICU personnel) may easily equal or exceed time lost in transportation, *and*
  - Problems in assuring reliability of results (quality control, uniform technique, calibration) as well as in care of equipment when testing is done by a large number of physicians and nurses who change with each shift
- Requirements for an emergency program in a centralized laboratory:
  - A centralized laboratory responsible for basic testing must have an emergency unit capable of providing fast service 24 hours a day.

  1. Organizational prerequisites:
     a) Constant 24-h on-call service
     b) Precise identification of specimens with notation of exact time
     c) Rapid, accurate communication of results:
        - Communication by telephone is time-saving and permits questions. Nevertheless, mistakes are common when information is passed on and documented in this fashion. Telephone conversations also cause loss of time for the laboratory technician. The telephone should never be the sole means of transmitting information.
        - Written findings should be sent by messenger, pneumatic tube, or teletype.
        - Direct transmission of data via computer is elaborate and expensive.
     d) Conscientious performance of checks for precision and accuracy

    e) Comparison of methods and results in routine and emergency laboratory facilities at frequent, regular intervals

    f) Thorough familiarization of medical technicians from the routine laboratory with procedures in the emergency unit

2. Personnel requirements for a large emergency laboratory (hospitals with more than 400 beds):
   - 2 or 3 medical technicians during normal working hours, as well as from 8 a.m. to 2 p.m. on Sundays and holidays
   - Constant availability of service at night

3. Equipment requirements for a large emergency laboratory (hospitals with more than 400 beds):
   - The emergency laboratory's equipment must be completely independent of that of the routine facility.
   - Automatic analyzers capable of running a certain selection of emergency tests have proved suitable.
   - The equipment may be varied according to the number of beds and demands placed on the laboratory.

- Acceptable organizational compromise:
  - Testing by the ICU laboratory: dipstick assays of urine and blood, blood gas analyses, osmometry, and oncometry
  - All other testing done by the central emergency laboratory
  - Findings to be reported to the ICU by telephone only when they exceed previously agreed-upon critical values; all other findings to be reported in writing only

Principle – Indications

- Identification and differentiation of pathogenic microorganisms and assessment of resistance to antibiotics in cases of manifest or suspected infection
- Recognition and differentiation of changes and shifts in the pathogen spectrum
  - in the same individual
  - with regard to potential cross infections within the ICU
- Identification and documentation of ICU-specific nosocomial pathogens (small space epidemiology).
- Routine hygiene checks of personnel and equipment on ICUs.
- Identification and differentiation of facultative pathogens as well, especially of saprophytic hitchhikers.
- Intensive care units have a unique constellation of microbiologic and hygiene problems, since infectious diseases as secondary conditions are very common. A clinically relevant infection may develop either from the patient's own germ reservoir (endogenous or due to autoinfection), or from ambient sources of contamination.
  Remember:
  The most important germ reservoir in the ICU is the severely ill, immunodeficient patient. The most important transmitter of infection is the personnel.
- Basic rules for avoidance of infectious complications:
  - Strict observance of rules by the entire personnel
  - Regular checks of hygienic conditions of the ICU and individual pieces of equipment (especially ventilating apparatus and nebulizers) in cooperation with the hospital's hygiene specialist
  - Prevention of infection of intravascular and bladder catheters by observing strict indications for placement, appropriate care of the catheters, hygienic handling of infusions, replacement of tubing systems for infusions at regular intervals (q 24 h)
  - Replacement of hose systems and humidifiers at regular intervals (at least q 24 h) for patients undergoing ventilation
  - Use of disposable equipment (also justified by the cost effectiveness ratio)
  - Preventive measures such as sterilization, disinfection, and wiping with disinfectant solution at regular intervals
  - Cooperation of clinicians, microbiologists, and hygiene experts

Microbiology and Hygiene Control

Equipment – Techniques

- Taking of specimens:
  - Tracheal secretions: sterile endotracheal suction with a special sampling tube containing a sputum trap interposed in the suction hose, suspension of the sample in fluid, attempt to quantify pathogens
  - Urine: puncture of the receptacle system at the site provided, following prior disinfection; refilling into a sterile tube
  - Wound secretions and drains: sterile sampling with swab from a special tube prefilled with transport medium (Results must be interpreted with caution, as tubing systems and wound surfaces are more likely to be colonized by foreign microorganisms than the hollow being drained).
  - Blood cultures, aerobic and anaerobic: sterile sampling in special tubes (Vacutainer) prefilled with culture medium
  - Immediate dispatchment of samples to the appropriate laboratory, as delays may falsify results
  - If anaerobic infection is suspected, use of appropriate special sampling sets
- Sampling intervals: For routine supervision of ventilated patients and those with urinary bladder catheters, bacteriology (pathogens and resistance) of urine and tracheal secretions should be done on admission of the patient to the ICU and at least once (preferably 2 or 3 times) a week thereafter.
- Evaluation of findings: All bacterial results must be interpreted in the context of the overall situation and clinical evidence of infection. Quantitative analysis of the microorganisms found considerably improves the relevance of results regarding contamination, infection, or therapeutic efficacy.

Documentation

- Findings must be recorded chronologically for each patient.
- Also desirable, and compulsory for large central units, is identification and analysis of the range of pathogens in the ICU as a whole. Only in this fashion is it possible to identify nosocomial microbes and determine their resistance spectrum.
- Supervision of microbiologic and hygienic surveys should be the responsibility of one individual.

Nursing Aspects

- Members of the nursing staff have the most frequent direct contact with the patient, and are therefore the greatest potential transmitters of infections. They are also responsible for inspection, maintenance, and daily availability of equipment. Nursing personnel must therefore be sufficiently well-trained to grasp the mental associations required for their work. Each ICU should have a firm supervisory regimen for all aspects of its function:
  - Establishing times for taking routine specimens
  - Assurance of prompt transportation
  - Establishing times and intervals for change of tubing systems and apparatus
  - Establishing precise intervals for disinfection, wiping with disinfectant, and change of linens
  - Change of smocks when changing to other patients or in other rooms (Overshoes are not a hygienic requirement.)
  - Disinfection of hands
  - Training in sterile suctioning technique and proper sampling of secretions

Central Venous Pressure

Principle

- Assessment of pressure in the valveless major intrathoracic venous system; best position is just distal to the junction of the superior vena cava and the right atrium

- The central venous pressure (CVP; normal range, 4–12 cm H_2O) depends on blood volume, functional competence of the right heart, intrathoracic pressure, and venous tone.

  1. Blood volume: CVP is proportionate to blood volume when the following, normal conditions prevail:
     - Functional competence of the right heart
     - Uncompromised pulmonary circulation
     - Normal, constant mean intrathoracic pressure
     - Normal venous tone

     If these conditions do not prevail, no inferences regarding changes of blood volume may be drawn from changes in central venous pressure.

  2. Functional competence of the right heart, e.g., in:
     - Myocardial failure, which causes venous pressure to rise above levels to be expected from the circulating blood volume alone
     - Pericardial tamponade or pericardial constriction, which raise CVP above levels due to circulating blood volume alone

  3. Compromised blood flow in the pulmonary circulation, e.g., in:
     - Pulmonary artery embolism, which causes CVP to rise above levels due to circulating blood volume alone

  4. Elevated intrathoracic pressure, e.g., in:
     - Positive-pressure ventilation, especially when the end-expiratory pressure is positive
     - Tension pneumothorax

  5. Enhanced venous tone:
     - Elevated venous tone (due to endogenous release of catecholamines, administration of vasopressor catecholamines, e.g., norepinephrine or dopamine) raises venous pressure above levels expected on the basis of blood volume alone.

- In manifest circulatory shock there is no correlation between blood volume and absolute CVP readings. CVP changes under such conditions are nevertheless an important basic variable in therapeutic administration of fluids (see pp. 67, 73, 132).

- Under certain conditions, CVP may serve as an indicator of the amount of extracellular fluid, i.e., as a measure of tissue turgor.
  1. CVP is less clearly correlated to the overall fluid balance than to blood volume, especially when changes occur slowly.
  2. CVP is an indicator of fluid homeostasis only if certain conditions are fulfilled:
     a) CVP must correlate to the blood volume (see above).
     b) Distribution of extracellular fluid between the intravascular (blood volume) and extravascular compartments must be normal, permitting blood volume to be regarded as a subcompartment of the extracellular compartment, and thus as reflecting changes in the extracellular fluid as a whole.
     Therefore, CVP reflects conditions in the fluid balance only when the following prerequisites for normal fluid distribution are met:
     – Normal oncotic plasma pressure
     – Normal hydrostatic capillary pressure
     – Normal capillary permeability
  3. Low oncotic plasma pressure, elevated capillary pressure, or enhanced permeability of the capillaries cause fluid to shift into the extracellular compartment or to become sequestered in a third compartment. This leads to hypovolemia and low CVP, despite normal or elevated total body water.

Indications

- Monitoring and identification of abnormal intravascular volume and disorders of fluid balance in severely ill patients.
- Monitoring of IV infusion therapy:
  – Maintenance of water and electrolyte homeostasis
  – IV alimentation
  – Forced diuresis
- Monitoring and control of volume replacement in:
  – Gastrointestinal hemorrhage
  – Acute abdomen
  – Shock
  – Acute renal failure
  – Extracorporeal hemodialysis, hemoperfusion
  – Mechanical ventilation

Equipment – Technique

- Assessment is usually by standpipe manometry. Readings are entered in a protocol or off-line in a computer-supported monitoring system:
  - If equipment is available, CVP may be measured by a pressure sensor, and the integrated results displayed and stored via TV monitor.
- As a rule, readings are taken with the patient in the flat supine position. Zero level is defined as $\frac{2}{5}$ the length of the anteroposterior sagittal thoracic diameter.
  - Readings may also be taken with the patient semierect or in lateral recumbent position.

    Zero level on the semierect patient: $\frac{2}{3}$ of the anteroposterior thoracic diameter at the level of the 4th intercostal space

    Zero level in lateral recumbent position: thoracic midline (sternum or vertebral spines)
- In PEEP (positive end-expiratory pressure)-ventilated patients, the effects of the elevated intrathoracic pressure must enter into interpretation of CVP data. It is not necessary to interrupt PEEP ventilation while measuring CVP if this is done.
- *Procedure:*
  - Adjust the standpipe to zero level (right atrium, see above).
  - Attach the central venous catheter to the tube system of the standpipe.
  - Take CVP readings (normal: 4–12 cm H_2O; definitely abnormal: less than 2 cm H_2O or above 14 cm H_2O).

Complications – Sources of Error

- Misinterpretation due to technical shortcomings:
  - False placement of the catheter tip
  - False adjustment of zero level
  - Kinking of the catheter
  - Clotting at the tip of the catheter
  Remember:
  Do not neglect to check catheter for patency and for fluctuations transmitted to the water column by due to pressure changes, pulse, and breathing excursions
  Do not take readings:
  - before equilibration of pressure.
  - when the patient is coughing or straining.
- Misinterpretation due to intellectual errors:
  - Deficient comprehension of the complex variables involved
  - Failure to consider technical sources of error in evaluation of elevated readings
  Remember:
  Normal CVP may vary widely, i.e., normal volumes may correspond to a wide range of pressure readings. Therefore, except for clear-cut deviations from the normal range, repeated measurements of CVP are more informative than individual readings. The following CVP changes do *not* reflect changes in volume and must be considered in interpreting readings:
  - Changes in position
  - Positive-pressure ventilation
  - Fluctuations of intrapleural pressure
  - Competence of the right heart
  - Obstruction of pulmonary vessels
  - Fluctuations in venous tone

Pulmonary Artery Catheterization

Principle

- Assessment of pulmonary artery and pulmonary capillary wedge pressure
- Determination of cardiac output
- Measurement of O_2 saturation of mixed venous blood

Indications

- Conditions in which catheterization of the pulmonary artery is indicated are:
  - Acute myocardial infarction
  - Protracted shock
  - Disorders in which the hemodynamic situation is difficult to evaluate, especially when sepsis is involved
  - Circulatory impairment during mechanical ventilation
  - Pulmonary edema of uncertain origin
  - Embolism of a pulmonary artery
  - Monitoring of therapy with large doses of cardiocirculatory drugs in critical situations
  - Therapy-resistant myocardial failure

Instruments

- Swan-Ganz balloon catheter
- Pressure transducer coupled to an electromanometer

Technique

- Following disinfection and local anesthesia of the skin, a suitable vein (basilic, external or internal jugular, subclavian, or femoral vein) is punctured or venous cutdown carried out.
- The Swan-Ganz catheter is introduced and advanced to the right atrium under guidance by observation of pressure changes.
- The catheter balloon is filled with about 1 mL of air.
- The catheter is further advanced to the pulmonary artery under pressure guidance.
- Position of the catheter tip is verified by roentgenography.
  Remember: In case of elevated pulmonary arterial pressure or markedly decreased cardiac output, advancement of the catheter under pressure guidance may be difficult. Advancement with fluoroscopic control is a useful alternative.

Recording
- Via electromanometer

Complications

- Perforation of the pulmonary artery: more common in elderly patients and in the presence of pulmonary hypertension, but rare on the whole

- Pulmonary infarction due to protracted occlusion of a branch of the pulmonary artery by the tip of the catheter or the inflated balloon
Remember:
Repeated verification of the catheter's position by observing pressure is mandatory.

- Knotting of the catheter

- Thrombophlebitis of long-residing catheters (more than 48 h), preventable by heparinization (p. 303) (Incidence of clinically apparent thrombosis is about 1%).

- Thrombotic occlusion of the catheter, rendering pressure measurement and irrigation of catheter impossible; removal of catheter mandatory
Prevention: Heparinization

- Cardiac arrhythmias: extrasystolic beats, bursts of ventricular extrasystole, ventricular tachycardia, ventricular fibrillation

- Infection and catheter sepsis (incidence reported in the literature: sepsis 0–10%, contamination of the catheter tip 15–20%)

Assessment of Cardiac Output

Indications

- Assessment of cardiac output (C.O.) is appropriate in:
  - Cardiogenic shock, septic shock
  - Severe left-sided myocardial failure
  - Pulmonary embolism
  - Circulatory impairment during mechanical ventilation
  - Monitoring of active cardiocirculatory drug therapy in critical cases

Instruments

- Swan-Ganz balloon catheter equipped with a thermistor tip
- C.O. thermodilution computer

Technique

- Puncture of a suitable vein (see p. 32).
- Introduction and advancement of the catheter into the pulmonary artery under roentgenographic or pressure-monitoring visualization (see p. 32).

Measurement

- Via C.O. computer coupled to the catheter; injection of 3.5 or 10 mL sterile saline with a temperature of 0–1°C (or 24°C) via the proximal lumen; automatic C.O. computer display of the measurement data

Sources of Error

- *Warming of the cold solution:* use of too warm a solution, or increase of its temperature within the apparatus due to technical delays
- *Respiration-dependent fluctuations of cardiac output,* particularly in deep spontaneous respiration and positive-pressure ventilation
- *Inappropriate position of the thermistor against a wall,* e.g., in the vicinity of the pulmonary valve, at the origin of a vessel, or in case of excessive peripheral advancement of the catheter
- *Intracardiac shunting,* especially from right to left, rendering measurements worthless by mixing and recirculating the blood

Complications

- Complications of C.O. determination are the same as those of pulmonary artery catheterization (see p. 33).

Noninvasive Peripheral Sphygmomanometry

- Conventional assessment of blood pressure via inflated cuff is the basic method in the ICU, as elsewhere.
- Potential sources of error:
  - Improperly calibrated sphygmomanometer
  - Tilting of mercury sphygmomanometer
  - Cuff too narrow (less than 40% of arm circumference) or too resilient
  - Improper application of cuff: too loose, so tight as to interfere with circulation, or too close to elbow
  - Improper positioning of arm: dependent position, failure to assure relaxation of arm
  - Inadequate pressure of pumped-up cuff
  - Stethoscope too far from brachial artery, or applied with too much pressure
  - Too rapid release of cuff pressure
  - Premature interruption of measurement, with risk of overlooking the so-called "auscultatory gap"
  - Repetition of measurement too soon or while arm is still congested
  - Sequelae to trauma or deformities of the arm
- Limitations of the method:
  Results may be unreliable in conditions with marked slowing of blood flow (particularly shock) or elevated peripheral resistance; readings tend to be lower than intravascular pressure.

Direct Arterial Sphygmomanometry

Indications

- Shock with undetectable blood pressure levels, particulary when peripheral resistance is known to be high (e.g., following administration of vasoconstrictive drugs)
- Monitoring of patients with fluctuating blood pressure (hemodynamic instability)

Equipment

- Plastic cannula with stylus, or percutaneous catheter (narrow-gauge Teflon catheter), electronic pressure sensor, pressure gauge and/or recording apparatus, disinfectant, local anesthetic, sterile cloth, sterile gloves, syringes

Techniques

- There are 2 methods:
  1. Puncture of an artery that is accessible to compression (radial, brachial, or femoral artery) by a plastic cannula containing a stylus; after removal of the stylus, connection of the system to the manometry equipment (pressure transducer, pressure gauge and/or recorder, TV display)
  2. Puncture of one of the above-mentioned arteries (preferably a femoral artery), and introduction of a narrow-gauge catheter
- Recording onto paper, if a paper scriber is available; otherwise, reading of measurement data from the manometer or TV screen

Complications

- Trauma to the artery with consequent hemorrhage
- Thrombosis with complete or partial occlusion of the artery
- Sepsis (incidence about 4%)

Intracorporeal Electrocardiography

Indications

- Rhythm disorders that elude evaluation by surface ECG:
  - Most frequently, when atrial activity is not evident
  - When the site of conduction block is unclear
  - In case of wide QRS complexes: to differentiate supraventricular beats with aberrant conduction from ventricular beats

Equipment

- Electrode-bearing catheter or esophageal leads
- ECG apparatus: 2- or multiple-channel recorder
- Amplifier with bandpass filter (40–500 Hz) for derivation of the His bundle electrogram

Techniques

- Recording of esophageal electrogram: A so-called esophageal lead is positioned 28–40 cm from the front teeth.
- Recording of the atrial electrogram: A catheter-borne electrode is advanced to the right atrium via a vein of the neck, arm, or groin, and position verified by roentgenography or by recording a typical atrial ECG.
- Recording of His bundle electrogram: A catheter is introduced via the right femoral vein. The tip bearing 2 or several electrodes is positioned above the tricuspid valve.

Recording:

- Esophageal electrogram: The intracorporeal lead is derived against a unipolar chest lead: The esophageal electrogram shows biphasic atrial deflections (+−).
- Atrial electrogram: In sinus rhythm, negative (−) potentials are seen in the high atrium, biphasic (+−) potentials in the intermediate atrium, and predominantly positive (+) potentials in the lower part of the atrium.
- Intracorporeal electrograms derived from the superior vena cava resemble aVR (augmented volt right arm), and those from the inferior vena cava resemble aVF (augmented volt foot) leads (paper transport speed 50 mm/s).
- His bundle electrogram: In sinus rhythm, an atrial wave (A wave), a His wave (H wave), and a ventricular potential (V wave) can be discerned (paper transport speed 50–100 mm/s).

Complications

- Esophageal ECG: trauma to the esophagus, triggering of vasovagal reflex (potential source of cardiac arrest)
- Intracardiac ECG: induction of arrhythmias (extrasystole, ventricular tachycardia, or even fibrillation); hazard of thrombosis of the catheterized vein when intracardiac ECG derivation is required over a period of days

Indications

- Monitoring of patients in cardiac emergencies, even after transfer from the cardiac ICU
- Identification of bradycardial and tachycardial rhythm disorders as related to syncope, vertigo, or palpitations
- Monitoring of antiarrhythmic drug therapy
- Observation of ST-segment levels in suspected Prinzmetal's angina
- Suspected intermittent malfunction of artificial pacemaker

Equipment

- Central monitoring unit with short- or long-term storage capability. Computer-supported evaluation of arrhythmias is optional.

Technique

- Skin over the manubrium sterni and the right anterior axillary line must be shaved and grease removed with an organic solvent (benzene).
  Adhesive electrodes are applied to the surface of the thorax and coupled to telemetry apparatus by cable leads.

Recording:
- Continuously via oscilloscope and magnetic tape

Indications

- Suspected pericardial effusions and/or tamponade
- Suspected pulmonary embolism
- Suspected bacterial endocarditis
- Suspected cardiac tumor
- Suspected aortic dissection
- Peripheral embolism (to elucidate the source, e.g., mitral stenosis, mitral valve prolapse, endocarditis, intraventricular thrombi)
- Acute regurgitation by aortic or mitral valve
- Malfunction of prosthetic heart valves
- Evaluation of ventricular function in suspected cardiogenic shock
- Suspected rupture of interventricular septum or papillary muscle
- Identification of atrial beats in tachycardia of obscure origin

Equipment

- Mobile units are preferable.
  - One-dimensional (M mode) visualization is no longer recommended.
  - Two-dimensional visualization by mechanical or electronic cross-sectional echocardiography reflects both pattern of movement and spatial orientation of heart structures.
  - Transesophageal echocardiography provides better visualization of the atria and the aortic and mitral valves, particularly in patients with pulmonary emphysema, in those undergoing ventilation, and when thoracic aortic dissection is suspected.
  - Contrast echocardiography permits identification of the direction of blood flow, which is useful when rupture of the interventricular septum or intracardial shunts are suspected.
  - Doppler echocardiography and color-coded Doppler echocardiography provide information on the direction and velocity of blood flow. They are used to elucidate suspected malfunction of artificial heart valves and to estimate the severity of stenoses.

Technique

- Localization of heart structures and major vessels by application of the transducer at specified precordial, subxiphoidal, and suprasternal sites, and by introduction of the transducer into the esophagus
- *Recording:* Polaroid film, x-ray film, video printer, or video tape
- Limitations: Obesity and pulmonary emphysema interfere with transthoracic sonography.
- *Likelihood of error is increased when:*
  - The patient has a condition that interferes with sonography.
  - The transducer is inappropriately placed.
  - The examining physician lacks experience.

Indications

The grounds for ultrasound echography of the abdomen may be related to either organs or symptoms.

- *Kidneys:*
  1. Oligoanuria: differentiation of postrenal, renal, and prerenal causes. Sonographically guided renal biopsy may be appropriate to identify the cause of acute renal failure of obscure origin.
  2. Elevated BUN: differentiation of chronic renal disease and acute renal failure; to rule out hydronephrosis
  3. Hematuria: differentiation of bladder vs. kidney tumors, stones, and glomerulonephritis
  4. Sonographic guidance in establishing a percutaneous pyelostomy
  5. Evaluation of bladder size prior to suprapubic puncture
- *Acute abdomen:*
  - Free fluid
  - Intestinal obstruction (fluid-filled intestinal loops with/without peristalsis)
  - Pancreatitis
  - Cholecystitis, cholangitis
  - Acute hydronephrosis
- *Hemoglobin decrement of obscure origin:*
  - Intraabdominal hemorrhage (one- or two-stage splenic rupture)
  - Blood/fluid in the gut
- *Fever of unknown origin:*
  - Hydro- or pyonephrosis
  - Abdominal abscess
- *Pancreas:*
  1. Acute pancreatitis:
     - Verification of diagnosis
     - Morphologic examination of pancreas and peripancreatic tissue
     - Etiology: biliary concrements, hepatosteatosis
     - Serial monitoring: pseudocysts, abscesses, hemorrhage
  2. Chronic pancreatitis:
     Recognition of biliary or intestinal obstruction
- *Lungs:*
  - Pleural effusions
  - Hemothorax
  - Verification of pneumothorax
  - Sonographic guidance of diagnostic or therapeutic pleurocentesis

- *Hepatobiliary ducts:*
  1. Cholestasis: differentiation of intrahepatic from extrahepatic-mechanical forms
  2. Assessment of organ sizes
  3. Evaluation of hepatic blood vessels:
     - Budd-Chiari syndrome
     - Portal hypertension
     - Septic thrombophlebitis
     - Acute hepatic congestion
  4. Gallstones, cholecystitis
- *Gastrointestinal tract:*
  - Fluid accumulation: hemorrhage, ileus, obstruction

Equipment

- Mobile unit with rapid-sequence B-imaging (real-time scanner), frequency 2–5 MHz
- Sonographically guided puncture requiring a specially constructed transducer

Indications

- *Arterial system:*
  - Identification and localization of peripheral artery obstructions
  - Differentiation of organic occlusion from vascular spasms (ergotism, Raynaud's syndrome)

    Accuracy of findings on extremity arteries exceeds 90%; diagnostic value of findings on the abdominal aorta, renal arteries, and visceral arteries is limited by the penetrating power.

    Accuracy in regions supplied by the common carotid artery is better than 90% in identification of high-grade stenosis or occlusion of extracranial portions of the carotid arteries.
  - Doppler sonography of the supratrochlear artery (an extracranial vessel that traverses the medial canthus and reflects conditions in the region supplied by the internal carotid artery), providing clues to cerebral ischemia in that area
- *Venous system:*
  - Doppler sonography in combination with compression and Valsalva maneuvers

    Iliac vein thrombosis can be identified with 90% accuracy.
  - Identification of thrombosis of the femoral and popliteal veins; noninvasive course monitoring during lytic therapy

Principle

- Taking roentgenograms under critical care conditions, particularly for radiographic evaluation of thoracic and abdominal organs. The quality of roentgenograms taken in bed is naturally not as good as that of those taken on a table or other support. Still, valid information may be obtained on the following:
  1. *Thorax:*
     - Verification of catheter or tube position
     - Alveolar and interstitial pulmonary changes, especially early signs of overinfusion and shock conditions
     - Inflammatory infiltrations
     - Complications, e.g., pneumothorax, hemothorax, and atelectasis
     - Cardiac size and configuration
     - Left-sided and right-sided heart failure
     - Effusions

     Remember:
     Except for check of position of catheter or tube, the above changes can often be verified only by serial pictures taken at intervals during the course.
  2. *Abdomen:*
     - Identification of free air
     - Identification of air-fluid levels
     - Toxic dilation of the colon
     - Opacities, densities

Indications

- Every ICU patient requires radiographic appraisal at certain intervals:
  - During mechanical ventilation: daily or every other day
  - Shock: daily
  - Hemodialysis, hemofiltration, hemoperfusion: before and after each session
  - Sepsis: daily or every other day
  - Following cardiopulmonary resuscitation: daily or every other day
  - Following aspiration: daily
  - Pneumonia: daily or every other day
  - Poisonings, especially with carbromal (chest and plain abdominal x-rays): on admission and after detoxification
  - Suspected perforation: ⎫
  - Suspected intestinal obstruction: ⎬ as soon as suspected

Remember:
Prompt radiographic verification of position of every vascular catheter and every thoracic drain as well as of corrections of position, is essential.

Equipment

- Mobile x-ray units with or without electric batteries are required for taking x-rays in bed.
- Units with 120–130 kV allow high-kV technique for chest x-rays, as well as filter techniques that permit better radiographic evaluation of the lungs.

Techniques

- Specially constructed beds equipped with cassette drawers that can be slid into proper position beneath the mattress facilitate optimum pictures without disturbing the patient. In the absence of this feature the film cassette may be inserted directly beneath the patient, with careful attention to proper supine positioning, reproduced exactly for each follow-up x-ray.
- Standardized film-focal length of 150 cm (provided the tube is powerful enough) assures comparability of serial follow-up x-rays.
- Exposure time and voltage should be kept as constant as possible in each control series.
- Simple chest films are taken in flat supine position.
- Plain abdominal films are taken in lateral recumbent position with a horizontal ray path; in case of carbromal poisoning, anteroposterior x-rays are acceptable.
- Brief exposure times are needed for mechanically ventilated patients and those with respiratory failure, who are unable to hold their breath. Ventilation with a respiratory bag is preferable, the patient's condition permitting.
- Monitor cables and tube clamps should be removed to the greatest possible extent, and chest x-rays taken during deep inspiration.

Documentation

- Each roentgenogram must bear the patient's name and birthdate, date the x-ray was taken, exposure time, voltage data, abbreviated description of ray path, and indication of sides.
- If it is not possible or (rarely) not necessary to take an x-ray for verification immediately after placement of a vascular catheter has been corrected, the shift must be indicated in centimeters on the original x-ray.

- A written report must be made on each x-ray. Precise descriptions of findings by both the radiologist and the clinician improve the usefulness of radiographic evidence.
- It is useful to keep the x-rays in the vicinity of the patient (inspection on bedside screens, if necessary on windows).

Complications

- Disconnection from ventilating apparatus when patient's position is altered
- Incidents related to intolerance of contrast medium

Nursing Aspects

- In addition to qualified x-ray technicians, assistance by nursing personnel is indispensable for good roentgenograms:
  - Assistance in positioning the patient
  - Covering the cassette with a cloth to protect it
  - Removal of cables and clamps
  - Assisting the patient in holding his breath (ventilation bag, appropriate adjustment of the ventilation apparatus)
  - Removal of bronchial secretions by suction prior to chest x-rays

Computerized Axial Tomography (CAT, CT)

Principle

- The attenuation of x-rays during passage through the body is measured in "layers" and related to the absorption capacity of water. By analyzing the stored measurement data, the computer is able to reconstruct an image based on density variations within the body under study. The density of certain structures may be enhanced by IV administration of an opaque medium, which permits better differentiation of normal and abnormal structures.

Indications

- For CT scanning, even critically ill patients must be transported to the machine. Still, since the information provided by this procedure is highly reliable, there are undisputed indications for it (within reasonable limits):
  1. Cranial CT:
     CT is appropriate in coma of obscure etiology when bedside examinations fail to clarify the cause. It permits identification and elucidation of:
     - Cerebral edema
     - Hemorrhage
     - Encephalomalacia (serial examinations)
     - Brain abscess
     - Craniocerebral trauma, sub- and epidural hematomas
     - Herpetic encephalitis (in some cases)
  2. Abdominal CT:
     Acute intraabdominal conditions that would normally mandate surgical intervention, but require particularly careful definition due to the vital risk and the hazards of surgery, justify CT of the abdomen. Abscesses, cysts, and necrosis, e.g., in pancreatitis or as postoperative complications, may be thusly identified. Echography should always precede CT scanning.

Preparation – Procedure
- Precautionary measures to insure respiratory and circulatory function during transportation and the examination itself:
  - Inspection of IV lines
  - Intubation if required
  - Vasoactive drug infusions in appropriate cases
  - Sedation of the patient
  - Attendance by a nurse familiar with the care of the patient

Therapeutic Intervention Scoring System (TISS)

Principle

- The severity of the course and the prognosis for critically ill patients in the ICU depend on the underlying condition and on complications, extent and number of disorders of vital functions, and type of intensive care required. TISS is an attempt at objective assessment of severity for purposes of classifying ICU patients by quantifying therapeutic intervention.

Procedure

- Each treatment procedure in intensive care is assigned a value of 1 to 4 points.
  It is assumed that the therapeutic procedures weighted with 4 points are used only in treatment of patients with the most severe conditions and courses.
- In this system of evaluation, the most critically ill of the patients requiring intensive therapy accrue 40–50 points (mean 43 ± 1.0 points, lethality 73%); patients requiring full intensive care amass 20–39 points (mean 23 ± 1 point, lethality 21%); patients in need of intensive monitoring only reach 10–19 points (mean 11 ± 1.7 points, lethality 15%).
- 4 points:
  - Cardiac arrest or electrical countershock within the past 48 h
  - Controlled ventilation with or without PEEP
  - Controlled ventilation with intermittent or continuous muscle relaxants
  - Balloon tamponade of esophageal varices
  - Continuous arterial infusions
  - Pulmonary artery catheter
  - Atrial and/or ventricular pacing
  - Hemodialysis in instable patients
  - Peritoneal dialysis
  - Induced hypothermia
  - Pressure-activated blood transfusions
  - G-suit
  - Intracranial pressure monitoring
  - Platelet transfusions
  - Intraaortic balloon assist (IABA)
  - Emergency operative procedures within the past 24 h
  - Lavage of acute gastrointestinal bleeding
  - Emergency endoscopy or bronchoscopy
  - Vasoactive drug infusion (more than 1)

Therapeutic Intervention Scoring System (TISS)

- 3 points:
  - Central IV hyperalimentation
  - Pacemaker on standby
  - Chest tubes
  - Intermittent mandatory ventilation (IMV) or assisted ventilation
  - Continuous positive end-expiratory pressure (CPAP)
  - Concentrated K^+ infusion via central catheter
  - Nasotracheal or orotracheal intubation
  - Blind intratracheal suction
  - Complete metabolic balance (frequent input and output)
  - Multiple ABG (arterial blood gas), bleeding, and/or STAT studies (more than 4/shift)
  - Frequent infusions of blood products (more than 5 units within 24 h)
  - Bolus IV injections (unscheduled)
  - Vasoactive drug infusion (1 drug)
  - Continuous antiarrhythmia infusions
  - Cardioversion for arrhythmia (not defibrillation)
  - Hypothermia blanket
  - Arterial line
  - Acute digitalization within the past 48 h
  - Assessment of cardiac output by any method
  - Active diuresis for fluid overload or cerebral edema
  - Active therapy for metabolic acidosis or alkalosis
  - Emergency thora-, para-, or pericardiocentesis
  - Active anticoagulation (initial 48 h)
  - Phlebotomy for volume overload
  - Coverage with more than 2 IV antibiotics
  - Treatment of seizures or metabolic encephalopathy within 48 h of onset
  - Complicated orthopedic traction
- 2 points:
  - CVP monitoring
  - 2 peripheral IV catheters
  - Hemodialysis – stable patient
  - Fresh tracheostomy (less than 48 h)
  - Spontaneous respiration via endotracheal tube or tracheostomy (T-piece or face mask)
  - GI (gastrointestinal) feedings
  - Replacement of excess fluid loss
  - Parenteral chemotherapy
  - Hourly neuro-vital signs
  - Infusions of pitressin IV
  - Multiple dressing changes

- 1 point:
  - ECG monitoring
  - Hourly vital signs
  - Single peripheral IV catheter
  - Chronic anticoagulation
  - Standard fluid intake and output (q 24 h)
  - STAT blood tests
  - Intermittent scheduled IV medications
  - Routine dressing changes
  - Standard orthopedic traction
  - Tracheostomy care
  - Decubitus ulcer
  - Urinary catheter
  - Supplemental O_2 (nasal or mask)
  - Antibiotics IV (2 or fewer)
  - Chest physiotherapy
  - Extensive irrigations, packings, or debridement of wounds, fistulas, or colostomies
  - GI decompression
  - Peripheral hyperalimentation / intralipid therapy

References:
Cullen DJ, et al., Crit Care Med 1974;2:57 (original description);
Keene AR, Cullen DJ, Crit Care Med 1983;11:1 (modification and commentary)

Acute Physiology and Chronic Health Evaluation (APACHE)

Principle

- APACHE is a system of objective assessment of severity of the condition of ICU patients. The objective is a prognostic stratification of critically ill patients based on the likelihood of lethal outcome. It is possible to assign patients to categories of different severity (thus having different prognoses), with a considerable degree of certainty. The prediction of outcome for individual patients is somewhat less reliable.

- The classification system is based on the sum of points assigned to deviations from normal of functional data gathered in the ICU during the acute stage (acute physiology score), and the patient's age and health prior to admission to the ICU (chronic health evaluation).

Procedure

- Functional data gathered in the acute phase within the first 24 hours following admission to the ICU are weighted with 0 to +4 points in ascending order of abnormality. Of the 34 parameters evaluated in the original version (APACHE I), only 14 are still included in the updated version (APACHE II, Tables **3a–3c**). New parameters are age and chronic general state of health. The sum of the points scored indicates the degree of severity and prognosis of the patient's present condition: The higher the score, the worse the prospects, i.e., the greater the lethality risk for his category (Fig. **3**).

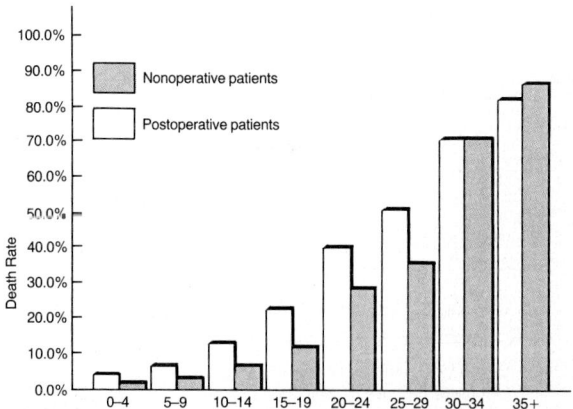

Fig. 3 APACHE II and hospital death: relationship between APACHE II scores and mortality among 5815 ICU admissions

Acute Physiology and Chronic Health Evaluation (APACHE)

Table **3a** The APACHE II Severity of Disease Classification System: Acute Physiology Score (APS)

Physiologic variable	High Abnormal Range		
	+ 4	+ 3	+ 2
Temperature (rectal, °C)	≥ 41	39–40.9	
Mean arterial pressure (mmHg)	≥ 160	130–159	110–129
Heart rate (ventricular response)	≥ 180	140–179	110–139
Respiratory rate (nonventilated or ventilated)	≥ 50	35–49	
Oxygenation: A–aDO$_2$ or PaO$_2$ (mmHg) a) FiO$_2 \geq 0{,}5$ A–aDO$_2$ b) FiO$_2 < 0{,}5$ PaO$_2$	≥ 500	350–499	200–349
Arterial pH	≥ 7.7	7.6–7.69	
Serum sodium (mmol/L)	≥ 180	160–179	155–159
Serum potassium (mmol/L)	≥ 7	6–6.9	
Serum creatinine (mg/100 mL) (Double point score for acute renal failure)	≥ 3.5	2–3.4	1.5–1.9
Hematocrit (%)	≥ 60		50–59.9
White blood count (per mm^3)	≥ 40		20–39.9
Glasgow Coma Score (GCS)	Score = 15 minus actual GCS		
Serum HCO$_3$ (venous, mmol/L) (not preferred; use if no ABGs)	≥ 52	41–51.9	

		Low Abnormal Range			
+ 1	0	+ 1	+ 2	+ 3	+ 4
38.5 ± 38.9	36–38.4	34–35.9	32–33.9	30–31.9	≤ 29.9
	70–109		50–69		≤ 49
	70–109		55–69	40–54	≤ 39
25–34	12–24	10–11	6–9		≤ 5
	< 200 > 70	61–70		55–60	< 55
7.5–7.59	7.33–7.49		7.25–7.32	7.15–7.24	< 7.15
150–154	130–149		120–129	111–119	≤ 110
5.5–5.9	3.5–5.4	3–3.4	2.5–2.9		< 2.5
	0.6–1.4		< 0.6		
46–49.9	30–45.9		20–29.9		< 20
15–19.9	3–14.9		1–2.9		< 1
32–40.9	22–31.9		18–21.9	15–17.9	< 15

Table **3b** Assignment of age points in the APACHE II Severity of Disease Classification System

Age (years)	Points
≤ 44	0
45–54	2
55–64	3
65–74	5
≥ 75	6

Table **3c** Weighting of chronic health condition in the APACHE II Severity of Disease Classification System

If the patient has a history of severe organ system insufficiency or is immunocompromised, assign points as follows:

a) For nonoperative or emergency postoperative patients   5 points
b) For elective postoperative patients   2 points

Definitions of Severe Organ Insufficiency and Compromise of the Immune System

Organ insufficiency or immunocompromised state must have been evident **prior** to this hospital admission and conform to the following criteria:

Liver:
Biopsy-proven cirrhosis and documented portal hypertension; episodes of past upper GI bleeding attributed to portal hypertension; or prior episodes of hepatic failure/encephalopathy/coma.

Cardiovascular:
New York Heart Association Class IV.

Respiratory:
Chronic restrictive, obstructive, or vascular disease resulting in severe exercise restriction, i.e., unable to climb stairs or perform household duties; or documented chronic hypoxia, hypercapnia, secondary polycythemia, severe pulmonary hypertension (over 40 mmHg), or respiratory dependency.

Renal:
Receiving chronic dialysis.

Immunocompromised:
The patient has received therapy that suppresses resistance to infection, e.g., immunosuppression, chemotherapy, radiation, long-term or recent high-dose steroids, or has a disease that is sufficiently advanced to suppress resistance to infection, e.g., leukemia, lymphoma, AIDS.

- The lethality risk for a given score depends on the patient's underlying disorder, which must therefore be drawn into consideration (e.g., the risk of lethality for patients with congestive heart failure who score 10–19 points is 13%, compared to 26% for patients in septic shock and having a similar numerical score). Prediction of lethal outcome vs. survival can be made with 85% accuracy.

Reference:
Knaus WA, et al., Crit Care Med 1985;13:818–829

- The purpose of intensive care medicine is the monitoring and treatment of patients with serious latent or overt disorders of vital functions. Intensive care means maintenance or restoration of vital functions by compensation of life-threatening functional deficiencies or replacement of ineffective organic functions until normal function returns ("therapeutic mandate of critical care medicine"). The notoriously poor outcome following organ failure, particularly that of several organs, has increasingly led to a shifting of the orientation of intensive medicine toward *preventing* overt organ failure ("preventive mandate of critical care medicine").

- Disorders of vital functions may occur as complications of widely varied acute illnesses, intoxications, or trauma, and are temporarily the major determinants of the course. Classification of pathologic conditions as "non-disease-specific, direct causes of death" or as "factors contributory to death" is referred to as the *thanatogenetic principle.*

- Any condition which experience has shown to be particularly conducive to acute disorders of vital functions and organ failure may be designated as a condition predisposing to life-threatening complications in the system of classification used in intensive care medicine.

- The best-studied predisposing condition is acute myocardial infarction. It is so often accompanied by acute life-threatening complications that all patients with fresh myocardial infarction should undergo intensive monitoring.

- Intensive monitoring is also necessary in patients with other underlying disorders that may precipitate acute life-threatening complications.

- Comatose or paralyzed patients are threatened additionally by serious sequelae that of themselves predispose to life-threatening complications that may interfere critically with subsequent rehabilitation or cause permanent damage.

- Medical disorders predisposing to such complications are listed in Table **4**.

Table **4**   Predisposing disorders

Acute myocardial infarction
Severe coronary artery occlusion and pre-infarction syndrome
Potentially fatal arrhythmias
Acute decompensation of myocardial failure
Hypertensive crisis
Massive pulmonary artery embolism

Sepsis

Acute abdomen
Acute hemorrhagic necrotizing pancreatitis
Peritonitis
Acute gastrointestinal hemorrhage
Acute hepatic failure
Severe gastroenterocolitis

Acute renal failure

Acute bronchopulmonary and pulmonary disease with respiratory failure

Acute disorders of hemostasis

Coma
Exogenous intoxication
Endocrine crises

Neuromuscular disorders with potential impairment of respiration
Status epilepticus
Subarachnoid hemorrhage with potential impairment of respiration
Severe alcoholic delirium
Apallic syndrome

Cardiac Arrest

Definition

- Sudden, unexpected loss of evidence of circulatory and respiratory activity and absence of central nervous functions

Etiology – Pathogenesis – Pathophysiology

- *Pathogenetic mechanism:*
  - Ventricular fibrillation
  - Asystole
  - Electromechanical dissociation
- *Most frequent causes:*
  a) Cardiac:
  - Coronary heart disease: usually history of infarction and recent infarction
  - Valvular defects: usually aortic defects
  - Cardiomyopathy: hypertrophic, dilating, restrictive
  - AV (atrioventricular) conduction disorders
  - Sick sinus syndrome
  - So-called "torsades de points" tachycardia (polymorphic ventricular tachycardia with periodic change of amplitude and direction of ventricular complexes due to QT syndrome, defined as prolonged QT interval after correction for frequency)
  b) Extracardiac:
  - Respiratory: airway obstruction, respiratory paralysis, severe hypoxia
  - Electrolyte and acid-base imbalance
  - Electrocution, severe hypothermia
  - Exogenous or endogenous poisoning
  - Hypersensitivity reactions

Diagnosis

- Loss of consciousness within 10–15 s
- Loss of muscular tone within 10–15 s
- Generalized seizures within 10–40 s
- Respiratory arrest or terminal gasping after 15–60 s
- Dilated pupils after 10–60 s
- *Findings:*
  1. Clinical: unconsciousness, apnea, pallor, dilated pupils, absence of pupillary reflexes, absence of carotid pulse
  2. ECG:
     - In case of ventricular fibrillation: high-frequency, deformed QRS complexes of nonuniform configuration
     - In atrial and ventricular asystole: no evidence of electrical activity

- In ventricular asystole due to 3rd degree AV conduction block: only P waves present, no QRS complexes
- In electromechanical dissociation: evidence of both atrial and ventricular action

Differential Diagnosis

- Collapse: carotid pulse still palpable, cardiac sounds audible, evidence of spontaneous respiration, patient responds when spoken to
- Syncope: brief loss of consciousness with or without cardiac arrest; spontaneously reversible with rapid recovery
- Coma: carotid pulse palpable, heartbeats audible, evidence of spontaneous respiration

Immediate Care

Simple, life-saving procedures
- Cardiopulmonary resuscitation with closed-chest cardiac compression (see p. 274):
  - 2 inflations (duration of insufflation 1–1.5 s)
  - Palpation of carotid pulse (5–10 s)
  - In absence of palpable pulse, initiation of cardiac massage:

One-rescuer method:
  - 15 compressions at a rate of 80–100/min
  - 2 inflations (duration 1–1.5 s)
  - 4 cycles of 15 compressions and 2 inflations
  - Palpation of carotid pulse (5 s)
  - If pulse not palpable, continuation of mechanical resuscitation: 15 compressions and 2 inflations per cycle

Two-rescuer method:
  - 5 compressions at a rate of 80–100/min.
  - Inflation of 1–1.5 s duration in a break between compressions
  - At least 10 cycles of 5 compressions and 1 ventilation each
  - Palpation of carotid pulse (5 s)
  - If pulse not palpable: continuation of mechanical resuscitation: 5 compressions and 1 ventilation per cycle
- Establishment of IV line: preferably in a large vein of the forearm or elbow
- Precordial thump only with ECG monitoring

Continuing Care

Extended life-saving procedures

- If cardiopulmonary resuscitation must be continued, treatment is directed at the underlying pathogenesis (ECG findings).

- Ventricular fibrillation and pulseless ventricular tachycardia: defibrillation with increasing energy, starting at 200–400 WS. If ineffective: epinephrine 0.5–1 mg IV, followed by renewed defibrillation with maximum energy. If this too is ineffective, repeat defibrillation, alternately with lidocaine (1 mg/kg IV), and possibly $NaHCO_3$ as well (1 meq/kg IV). Once sinus rhythm has been restored: lidocaine drip (2–4 mg/min.) as a preventive measure.

- Ventricular tachycardia with palpable carotid pulse:
  - Patient unstable (thoracic pain, dyspnea, systolic pressure ≤90 mmHg, congestive heart failure, myocardial infarction): sedation and cardioversion, starting at 50 WS and proceeding to a maximum of 400 WS. If unsuccessful: lidocaine 1 mg/kg IV and repeat cardioversion. If ventricular tachycardia persists: administration of a class IA or IC antiarrhythmic drug (see p. 291) before repeating cardioversion
  - Patient stable: lidocaine 1 mg/kg IV; if ineffective, lidocaine 0.5 mg/kg IV q 8 min up to a total of 3 mg/kg. If ventricular tachycardia still persists: IV administration of a class 1A or 1C antiarrhythmic drug (see p. 291); if ineffective, cardioversion as for unstable patients.

- Asystole: epinephrine 0.5–1 mg IV, and intratracheal intubation if feasible. If asystole persists, administration of atropine 1 mg IV, and possibly $NaHCO_3$.
  Extracardiac sources of electromechanical dissociation, e.g., hypovolemia, pericardiac tamponade, tension pneumothorax, and pulmonary embolism, must be ruled out.

Prognosis

- Very serious. Unfavorable signs:
  - Electromechanical dissociation
  - Asystole
  - Preexisting heart damage
  - No acute myocardial infarction
  - Interval of more than 5 minutes elapsed before cardiopulmonary resuscitation is initiated

Definition

- Conditions involving cardiocirculatory failure with inadequate perfusion of peripheral tissues
- Classification:
  - Volume depletion shock
  - Cardiogenic shock
  - Septic shock
  - Anaphylactic shock
- The early, hyperdynamic phase of septic shock occupies a special category because of its etiology and symptoms (see p. 72).

Pathophysiology

- Three main causative mechanisms:
  - Reduction of circulating blood volume
  - Impairment of cardiac performance
  - Peripheral vascular failure
- Consequences: drop of cardiac output and blood pressure, centralization of blood flow, hypoxia with metabolic acidosis and intracellular metabolic disorders; disseminated intravascular coagulation (DIC)
- Shock due to overdosage of hypnotic drugs involves the entire spectrum of shock-producing factors: hypovolemia due to lack of fluid intake, sequestration of fluid in cutaneous tissue and muscle, and frequently vomiting; toxic impairment of cardiac performance; impairment of central and peripheral mechanisms governing circulation

Diagnosis

- Signs of illness:
  - Tachycardia
  - Arterial hypotension with narrow blood pressure amplitude
  - Cold, clammy, pallid-cyanotic, marbled skin (exception: warm, dry skin in septic shock)
  - Oliguria or anuria
  - Dyspnea
  - Anxiety, motoric unrest or impaired consciousness
- *Findings:*
  1. Clinical:
     - Peripheral circulation (hue, dampness, and temperature of skin, return of color to compressed nail base)
     - Other skin alterations (urticaria, hematomas)

63

– Turgor of neck veins (in horizontal supine position and with trunk inclined at a 45° angle)
– Cardiopulmonary function
– Urinary output
– Level of consciousness
2. Laboratory and technical:
   – Hb (hemoglobin), Hct (hematocrit), WBC (white blood count), platelet count, Quick's test, PTT, thrombin time, blood type
   – Sodium, potassium, creatinine, BUN, blood sugar, CK, GOT (glutamate-oxalate transferase), GPT (glutamate-pyruvate transferase)
   – pH, pCO_2, standard bicarbonate, base deficit in arterial blood
   – Lactic acid
   – Osmolality
   – Blood cultures (optional)
   – ECG
   – Chest x-ray
   – Central venous pressure, pulmonary artery catheter (optional)

Differential Diagnosis

• Collapse: no evidence of impaired perfusion of tissue
• Special types of shock, depending on the cause

Immediate Care

• Position: Flat supine, except in cardiogenic shock (head and chest elevated, legs lowered)
• Sedation and pain relief with diazepam (5–10 mg IV) or morphine (5–10 mg IV), if required. Keep individual doses small, and repeat as necessary
• IV line and administration of fluids:
   – Initial fluid expansion in the form of colloidal volume expanders or balanced electrolyte solutions
   – Immediate fluid volume replacement is always indicated in the absence of signs of decompensated heart failure (congested neck veins, orthopnea, rales over both lung bases).
• Compensation of respiratory failure:
   – Oxygen via nasal catheter (2–6 L/min) or mask (6–10 L/min)
   – Intubation and artificial ventilation in case of unconsciousness or protracted shock
• Correction of metabolic acidosis is indicated when pH is below 7.3 or base deficit exceeds 10 mmol/L.

Solutions:
– Bicarbonate. Dosage:
  meq $NaHCO_3$ = negative base excess $\times$ 0.3 $\times$ kg BW. If the
  calculated total amount exceeds 200 mEg, one-half should be
  given, and blood gases analyzed 2 hours later. Sodium content
  must be considered in patients with myocardial failure!
– THAM (tris-hydroxylmethyl aminomethane): sodium-free; preferable if sodium intake must be restricted
  Dosage: mL 0.3 molar THAM = neg. base excess $\times$ kg BW

Continuing Care

• Prerequisite for definitive therapy is more precise identification of
  the type of shock.
• Monitoring of the following parameters is mandatory:
  – Heart rate and rhythm (ECG, rhythm monitoring)
  – Arterial blood pressure (invasive or noninvasive)
  – CVP
  – Respiratory rate
  – Arterial blood gas analysis
  – Urine output
  – Level of consciousness
• Optional monitoring:
  – Pulmonary artery pressure
  – Cardiac output
  – Blood volume
  – Skin temperature

Complications

• Residual organ damage once shock has been overcome:
  – Acute renal failure
  – ARDS (adult respiratory distress syndrome)
  – Shock liver
• Disseminated intravascular coagulation

Hypovolemic Shock

Definition

- Acute circulatory failure consequent upon loss of blood, plasma, or water and electrolytes

Etiology – Pathogenesis

- Sources:
  1. Blood loss (hemorrhagic shock)
     - External bleeding: trauma to large vessels, gastrointestinal hemorrhage (bleeding esophageal varices, ulcers, erosions, diverticula, neoplasms), pulmonary hemorrhage (thoracic trauma, injury to the lungs, pulmonary tuberculosis, tumors), renal and/or vesical hemorrhage (tumors, prostate resection), female genital tract (miscarriage, postpartum hemorrhage)
     - Internal bleeding: retroperitoneal hemorrhage (ruptured abdominal aneurysm, hemorrhagic pancreatitis), intra-peritoneal hemorrhage (ruptured spleen or liver, infarcted or strangulated intestine, ectopic pregnancy), soft-tissue bleeding (trauma to muscle, fracture hematomas), ruptured aneurysms
     - Bleeding at diverse sites due to overdose of anticoagulants or hemorrhagic diathesis
  2. Losses of plasma, water, and electrolytes:
     a) External loss of fluid:
        - Gastrointestinal: massive vomiting, diarrhea, fistulas, post-surgical drainage
     b) Internal loss of fluid:
        - Blunt trauma, burns, peritonitis, pancreatitis, ileus

Diagnosis

- Clinical signs:
  a) Collapse of superficial veins
  b) Generalized shock symptoms
  c) Signs of hypovolemia, according to volume lost:
     - *Loss of about 10–25%:*
       Mild signs of peripheral vasoconstriction, mild tachycardia, blood pressure normal or slightly lowered
     - *Loss of about 25–30%:*
       Tachycardia 100–120/min, reduced pulse amplitude, systolic blood pressure 90–100 mHg, restlestness, pallor, sweating, oliguria
     - *Loss of about 35–50%:*
       Tachycardia exceeding 120/min, systolic blood pressure below 60 mmHg, clouded consciousness, pallor, very cold extremities, anuria

- Emergency history:
  - Thoracic pain, expectoration of blood
  - Abdominal pain, melena, hematemesis
  - Diarrhea, vomiting
  - Last menstrual period
  - Clotting disorders, anticoagulant drugs, trauma
- *Findings:*
  1. Clinical:
     - Inspection, auscultation, and palpation of thorax and abdomen
     - Palpation and auscultation of the abdominal aorta and the large peripheral vessels
     - Rectal digital palpation
  2. Laboratory:
     - Hb and Hct: information on blood loss to be provided only after several hours have elapsed
     - Serum amylase and lipase
     - Coagulation parameters
     - Chest and plain abdominal x-rays
     - Abdominal sonography

Immediate Care

- Positioning
  Shock: supine, horizontal or tilted with head and trunk lowered
- Volume replacement:
  - Blood loss in excess of 30%: blood and plasma (or colloid plasma expander solutions, provided coagulation is not impaired) in 1:1 ratio. When total replacement volume exceeds 4000 mL, the ratio should be 2:1.
    Remember:
    Acute, severe hemorrhaging may require simultaneous replacement via several lines, and infusion of fluid under pressure.
  - Blood loss below 30% of blood volume: plasma or colloid plasma substitutes
  - Loss of plasma, water, and electrolytes: lost volume to be estimated on the basis of clinical evidence
  - Volume replacement: initially with plasma or colloid plasma extenders to refill the intravascular space. Once the circulating blood volume is stabilized, administration of balanced electrolyte solutions to normalize the extracellular fluid. CVP should level off at 6–10 cm H_2O.

- Correction of acidosis:
  pH below 7.3 and base deficit exceeding -10 mEq/L: $NaHCO_3$ or THAM solution.
  Remember:
  Vasoconstrictive drugs are absolutely contraindicated, since they lead to further impairment of peripheral circulation.

Continuing Care

- Continuation of volume replacement under control of:
  - CVP (minimum 4 cm H_2O, optimum 8–10 cm H_2O, maximum 12–14 cm H_2O)
  - Urine output (minimum 40 mL/h)
  - Peripheral circulation (appearance of skin, capillary refilling time, arterial blood pressure amplitude, heartrate)
  - Hematocrit (minimum 30 vol.%, optimum 35 vol.%)
- Treatment of the underlying disorder: definitive hemostasis required for hemorrhagic shock
- Monitoring of renal function: Urine output, serum creatinine, creatinine clearance (particularly if serum creatinine is normal), U/P_{osm}
- Monitoring of respiration and blood gases

Definition

- Acute circulatory failure due to inadequate cardiac pump performance

Etiology – Pathogenesis

- Causes:
  - Loss of contractile muscle: myocardial infarction, myocarditis
  - Acute rupture of interventricular septum or rupture of papillary
    muscle avulsion due to myocardial infarction
  - Decompensated valvular defects: chronic and acute (resulting
    from bacterial endocarditis or myocardial infarction)
  - Acute obstruction of pulmonary circulation: pulmonary embol-
    ism, intracardiac thrombi, heart tumors
  - Pericardial tamponade
  - Tachyarrhythmia

Diagnosis

- Symptoms: Triad:
  - Signs of shock with decreased blood pressure, usually to below
    90 mmHg (systolic)
  - Tachycardia: may be absent in inferior infarction
  - Oliguria
- *Findings:*
  1. Clinical: signs of heart failure (gallop rhythm, pulmonary rales)
     Remember:
     Complications of myocardial infarction: ruptured ventricular
     septum and for papillary muscle, pericarditis
     Special situation: in inferior myocardial infarction involving the
     right ventricle, heart rate usually not accelerated (2nd or 3rd
     degree AV block often present); signs right ventricular failure,
     lungs unremarkable
  2. Laboratory: CK, CK-MB, GOT
  3. ECG: signs of myocardial infarction (usually extensive anterior
     infarction; in inferior infarction involving the right ventricle: ST
     elevation in V_4R); arrhythmia
  4. Pulmonary arterial (PA) catheterization, thermodilution: car-
     diac output diminished (cardiac index below $2.2\,L\cdot min^{-1}\cdot m^2$),
     filling pressure in excess of 20 mmHg (right ventricular infarc-
     tion: elevated right atrial pressure)
  5. Echocardiography: impaired contractility, left ventricle usually
     enlarged, pulmonary artery dilated; possibly: valve leaflet altera-
     tions with regurgitation, impaired right ventricular contractility,
     interventricular shunt
  6. Chest x-ray: pulmonary congestion

Cardiogenic Shock

Differential Diagnosis

- Myocardial infarction plus hypovolemia: similar clinical symptoms, but with diminished filling pressure on PA manometry
- Other types of shock: filling pressure not elevated

Immediate Care

- Positioning: slight elevation of head and chest
- IV access line: cautious administration of fluid (250 mL/30 min)
- Analgesia: morphine 3–5 mg IV, if necessary repeated at 5-min intervals; combine with atropine if heartrate less than 60 bpm
- Oxygen: nasal tube 2–6 L/min, mask 6–10 L/min
- If systolic pressure is below 90 mmHg: dopamine until hemodynamic situation can be controlled in the ICU

Continuing Care

- Hemodynamic control of therapy by PA catheter:
  1. Reduction of elevated filling pressure to about 18 mmHg by nitroglycerin or sodium nitroprusside
  2. If response is unsatisfactory, administration of catecholamines: dobutamine (if blood pressure is still adequate) or dopamine (in event of hypotension: combined with nitroglycerin or dobutamine)
  3. Specific therapy:
     - Acute myocardial infarction: intracoronary thrombolysis and percutaneous transluminal Coronary angioplasty
     - Acute inferior infarction with right ventricular involvement: augmentation of right ventricular filling pressure (by more than 10 mmHg) by administration of fluid (Caution! Drugs that may reduce the preload are contraindicated), and acceleration of heartrate by atrial pacing (sequential stimulation in 3rd degree AV block)
     - Rupture of interventricular septum or papillary muscle rupture with acute regurgitation consequent upon myocardial infarction: sodium nitroprusside, early surgical intervention
     - Pulmonary embolism: embolectomy or fibrinolysis
     - Pericardial tamponade: pericardiocentesis
     - Cardiac tachyarrhythmia: antiarrhythmic drugs, electrostimulation, cardioversion

Prognosis

- Favorable only if the source is amenable to treatment (e.g., cardiac arrhythmias, pericardial effusions, emergency heart surgery)
- Unfavorable if the source cannot be eliminated (e.g., myocardial infarction)

Definition

- Shock in infections by gram-negative and gram-positive bacteria, less often by viruses, Rickettsia, parasites, or fungi

Etiology – Pathophysiology – Pathogenesis

- Predisposing factors:
  Urinary tract infections, biliary tract disorders, pneumonia, or peritonitis involving bacteremia; septic abortion, postpartum complications, disorders involving immunosuppression
- Most frequently encountered pathogens:
  - Gram-negative bacteria:
    E. coli, Klebsiella sp., Proteus, Pseudomonas aeruginosa, Aerobacter aerogenes, meningococci
  - Gram-positive bacteria:
    Staphylococcus aureus, Pneumococcus, Streptococcus haemolyticus
- Pathophysiology:
  - Early stages: hyperdynamic shock with warm, dry skin, respiratory alkalosis, increased cardiac output, decreased peripheral vascular resistance, normal or elevated CVP, and normal left-ventricular filling pressure
  - Later course: potential transition to hypodynamic state with cold, cyanotic, poorly perfused skin, metabolic acidosis, decreased cardiac output, elevated peripheral vascular resistance, diminished circulating blood volume, and propensity for disseminated intravascular clotting

Diagnosis

- Signs of illness:
  - Symptoms of bacterial infection (fever, chills)
  - Hyperventilation
  - Impaired overall condition
  - Confusion, signs of delirium, impairment of consciousness without apparent cause
  - Factors predisposing to septic shock: immediate postoperative period, indwelling urinary bladder catheter, indwelling IV line, tracheostomy, diabetes mellitus, liver cirrhosis, burns, malignancies, leukemia, agranulocytosis, therapy with corticosteroids or cytotoxic drugs

- *Findings:*
  1. Clinical: evidence of shock and signs of sepsis (fever, bacterial infection)
  2. Laboratory:
     - Blood count: leucocytosis or leukopenia, but with shift to the left, thrombocytopenia, hypophosphatemia
     - Bacteriology with resistance assessment of blood, urine, sputum, and stool or wound secretions in appropriate cases
     - Clotting studies: in case of disseminated intravascular coagulation: depression of thrombocytes, fibrinogen, clotting factors II, V, and X; enhancement of fibrinogen split products, and reduction of prekallikrein in plasma

Immediate Care

- Flat, recumbent positioning
- Placement of an IV line:
  - Volume replacement: plasma or dextran solution, blood transfusion only in case of blood loss. CVP should not exceed 14 cm H_2O.
  - Provide for ventilation (check that the airways are cleared, administration of O_2 4–6 L/min).
  - Correct metabolic acidosis.

Continuing Care

- Antibiotics:
  - Known pathogen: appropriate bactericidal antibiotics IV (resistance testing)
  - Unknown pathogen: combination of a bactericidal antibiotic with an aminoglycoside and an antibiotic that is effective against anaerobic microbes.
- Hemodynamically controlled volume replacement ("volume challenging"): volume replacement 250 mL/15 min, provided CVP is less than 14 cm H_2O and does not increase by more than 5 cm H_2O per volume/time unit; adjustment of PA pressure to 16–18 mmHg
- Corticosteroids: in the event that peripheral circulation is still poor after volume replacement: methylprednisolone 30 mg/kg IV, followed by 2 g q 6 h for 48 h, or dexamethasone 40 mg IV, followed by 20–40 mg q 4–6 h
  Duration of corticosteroid therapy: 24–72 h
- Heparin 1000 U/h continuous drip

- Vasoactive medication: if the basic treatment (volume replacement, O_2, compensation of acidosis) fails to control shock:
  - Dopamine in increasing dosage from 200–400–600 µg/min. If the effect on cardiac output even at this dosage is inadequate:
  - Addition of dobutamine in incremented dosage steps of 200–400–600 µg/min. If the circulation still remains unstable:
  - Increase of the combined dopamine-dobutamine dosage to 800–1000 µg/min, depending on the effect
    If even this dosage fails to increase systolic blood pressure to at least 100 mmHg, or if blood pressure is maintained by marked tachycardia (over 120–130 bpm):
  - Addition of norepinephrine in dosage increments of 10–100 µg/min
- Surgical measures: once the circulation is stable, surgical treatment of localized sites of infection
  Remember:
  If the focus of infection is not eradicated, definitive stabilization of a septic patient is impossible. Intensive therapy can only provide the framework for management of the septic focus. Any measures serving to combat the septic focus are part of definitive intensive therapy.

Prognosis

- Serious; very grave if:
  - the source of infection cannot be eliminated;
  - malignancy is the basic condition;
  - persistent or progressive hyperlactacidemia is present;
  - multiple organ complications occur (acute renal failure, acute respiratory failure, gastrointestinal hemorrhaging, acute hepatic failure).

Definition

- Shock due to a severe systemic hypersensitivity reaction of the immediate type

Etiology – Pathogenesis

- Triggering antigens:
  - Drugs:
    Antibiotics, local anesthetics, radiographic contrast media containing iodine, colloidal volume replacement solutions
  - Foreign proteins and polysaccharides:
    insect or snake venoms, sera, vaccines, organ extracts, solutions of allergens for desensitization
- Systemic antigen-antibody reactions cause liberation of vasoactive substances (histamine, serotonin, bradykinin), which produce acute vascular dilation (especially of the veins) and consequent reduction of the return of venous blood to the heart, cardiac output, and arterial blood pressure. Plasma loss may occur due to enhanced permeability of the vessels.

Diagnosis

- *Symptoms:*
  Seconds or minutes after exposure to the allergen, the following symptoms may develop, depending on the severity:
  1. Cutaneous reactions: flush, erythema, urticaria, edema. Generalized symptoms: pruritus, agitation, dizziness, headache, tremor
  2. Hemodynamic reactions:
     - Heartrate increase of more than 20 bpm
     - Decrement of systemic blood pressure by more than 20 mmHg
     Gastrointestinal symptoms: nausea, vomiting, diarrhea, abdominal pain
  3. Shock symptoms with hypotension: impaired consciousness, severe bronchoconstriction
  4. Vasomotor and respiratory collapse
- *Findings:*
  1. Clinical: mucosal edema, bronchospasms, impaired respiration, skin changes
  2. Laboratory: leukopenia, thrombopenia

Anaphylactic Shock

Immediate Care

- Epinephrine 0.1 mg (1 mL of a 1-mg ampule of epinephrine diluted in 10 mL saline IV; may be repeated q 5–10 min
- Corticosteroids, e.g., methylprednisolone 250 mg IV
- Volume replacement infusions (e.g., 5% human albumin or plasma protein solution). Colloid volume replacement solutions are contraindicated due to their potential allergenic effects
- Antihistamines (e.g., diphenhydramine 25–50 mg IV)
- Clear airways for ventilation, in the event of laryngeal edema: intubation or tracheotomy
- Occasionally required in case of severe, persistent bronchial spasms: theophylline – ethylene diamine (aminophylline) 6 mg/kg as slow (10–20 min) IV drip

Continuing Care

- Volume replacement (see First Aid)
- Epinephrine as continuous IV drip if hypotension persists after volume replacement (dosage depends on the effect). In case of tachycardia it may be combined with norepinephrine 1–10 µg/min IV drip
- After resolution of shock symptoms, corticosteroids and antihistamines should be continued for 2 days

Complications

- Bronchial spasms
- Laryngeal edema
- Supraventricular and ventricular rhythm disorders
- Circulatory collapse

Prognosis

- The earlier specific treatment is initiated, the better. Once signs of shock have resolved, the prognosis is favorable.

Definition

- Congestive heart failure that fails to respond to conventional therapy (heart glycosides, diuretics) is referred to as therapy-refractory.

Etiology – Pathogenesis – Pathophysiology

- *Causes:*
  - Diseases of heart muscle: dilated cardiomyopathies
  - Coronary heart disease: so-called ischemic cardiomyopathy
  - Valvular disease: usually combined mitral and aortic defects
- *Pathophysiology:*
  Heart performance severely impaired, cardiac function curve flattened; consequent signs of congestion and reduced cardiac output

Diagnosis

- *Symptoms:*
  1. Signs of congestion:
     - Pulmonary circulation: orthopnea, resting dyspnea
     - Systemic circulation: congestion of neck veins, edema, ascites
  2. Signs of reduced cardiac output: fatigue, weakness, somnolence
- *Findings:*
  1. Clinical:
     - Cyanosis
     - Congestion of neck veins, edema, (occasionally) ascites
     - Hepatomegaly
     - Signs of tricuspid regurgitation (optional)
     - Moist rales over the bases of both lungs
     - Pleural effusions (optional)
  2. Hemodynamics: cardiac index decreased (usually to less than 2.5 L/min/m^2), left ventricular filling pressure elevated (usually to above 15 mmHg)
  3. Echocardiography: enlargement of both ventricles, reduced excursion of heart walls; valvular alterations in some conditions
  4. ECG: nonspecific
- *Differential diagnosis:*
  Other conditions involving edema (hepatic cirrhosis, chronic renal disease, protein-losing enteropathy); other signs of heart disease are lacking in these conditions
  Constrictive pericarditis

Therapy – Refractory Heart Failure

Immediate Care

- Positioning of patient with head and thorax elevated, legs lowered
- Oxygen administration: as required
- Diuretics: furosemide 20–40 mg IV

Continuing Care

- Strict restriction of sodium and fluids
- Drainage of effusions: pleurocentesis, possibly paracentesis
- Diuretics: furosemide 20–80 mg IV, combined with potassium-sparing diuretics (spironolactone, triamterene, amyloride) as required
- Sympathomimetic drugs: dobutamine (Dobutrex) drip for 2–7 days Amrinone (Innocor) drip for up to 14 days
- Vasodilating agents: drips: nitrates (e.g., nitroglycerin 5–100 µg/kg/min), sodium nitroprusside 0,5–8 µg/kg/min. Orally: prazosin up to 30 mg/day, nitrates (isosorbide dinitrate, max. 480 mg/day) combined with hydralazine, max. 300–450 mg/day; exceptional cases may require 2000 mg/day; ACE inhibitors (captopril, enalapril)
- Antiarrhythmic agents: as required

Complications

- Cardiac arrest due to ventricular fibrillation or primary asystole
- Phlebothrombosis, pulmonary embolism
- Hypostatic pneumonia

Prognosis

- Usually unfavorable, since the condition is the end stage of chronic heart disease; better if the basic heart condition can be improved or eliminated by surgery (acquired valvular disease, ventricular aneurysm)

Definition

- Effusion of fluid from the pulmonary capillaries into the interstitial spaces (interstitial pulmonary edema) and subsequently into the alveolar spaces (alveolar pulmonary edema) due to elevated pulmonary venous pressure

Etiology

- Acute left-sided heart failure: coronary heart disease, valvular defects, arterial hypertension, bradycardial or tachycardic arrhythmias, dilated cardiomyopathy
- Mitral valve obstruction: mitral stenosis, atrial myxoma

Diagnosis

- *Symptoms:* Dyspnea of increasing acuteness, with anxiety, cough, and expectoration of watery, reddish, foamy sputum
- *Findings:*
  1. Clinical:
     - Central cyanosis; audible, bubbly respiratory sounds
     - Moist, nontympanic to tympanic rales, initially over the lung bases, then ascending rapidly; occasionally dry rales (concomitant bronchospasm)
     - Cool, moist skin
     - Shock symptoms (optional)
     - 3rd heart sound, usually tachycardia, heart murmurs (in case of valvular defects that place strain on the left heart)
  2. ECG: sinus rhythm with signs of left atrial enlargement or atrial fibrillation, depending on the underlying disorder: signs of infarction, left ventricular hypertrophy, arrhythmias
  3. Chest x-ray:
     - Usually symmetrical hilar opacities with signs of pulmonary congestion
  4. Laboratory:
     - Arterial blood gas analysis: pO_2 reduced, pCO_2 initially reduced; development hypercapnia later in half of all cases
     - Cardiospecific enzymes elevated in case of infarction
  5. PA catheterization:
     PA and PWA (pulmonary wedge arterial) pressures elevated
  6. Echocardiography:
     Depending on the underlying disorder, signs of valvular defects, wall hypertrophy (hypertension), segmental wall motion abnormality (coronary heart disease)

Acute Pulmonary Edema

Differential Diagnosis

- Bronchial asthma: dry rales, signs of left heart failure not predominant, no mitral stenosis; on x-ray: lungs overfilled with air; no elevation of cardiospecific enzymes
- Pulmonary embolism: pain, signs of strain on right heart, but not on left heart

Immediate Care

- Positioning: head and thorax elevated, legs lowered
- Nitroglycerin sublingually 0.8–1.6 mg at intervals of 5–10 min
- Diuretics: furosemide (Lasix) 40–80 mg IV
- Sedatives: morphine 3–5 mg IV (may be repeated at 5-min intervals)
- Oxygen: 6–10 L/min via mask

Continuing Care

- Vasodilating agents (nitroglycerin or sodium nitroprusside) as continuous IV drip
- Aminophylline if dry rales persist
- If pulmonary edema is due to tachycardia: cardioversion or intracardiac pacing; in case of absolute tachyarrhythmia: digoxin 0.25–0.5 mg IV
- Antihypertensive drugs in event of hypertensive crisis
- Intubation and positive-pressure ventilation in severe pulmonary edema or deterioration during first aid
- Application of tourniquets to lower extremities (= noninvasive phlebotomy) or invasive phlebotomy (only in extreme situations)

Complications

- Death from asystole or ventricular fibrillation

Prognosis

- Grave; depends on basic condition: very poor in coronary heart disease and congestive cardiomyopathy, but better in case of arterial hypertension or valvular defects

Definition

- Impairment of diastolic filling of the heart caused by increased pressure within the pericardium due to accumulation of fluid

Etiology – Pathogenesis – Pathophysiology

- *Pathophysiology:*
  - Consequent upon the reduced cardiac filling, end-diastolic ventricular volume and stroke volume are also lessened. Cardiac output and blood pressure remain normal for awhile, thanks to compensation mechanisms. Once the increase in end-diastolic pressure reaches a critical level, however, cardiac output and blood pressure decrease abruptly (cardiac tamponade).
- Hemodynamic effects depend on:
  - Amount of fluid in the pericardium
  - Rapidity of fluid accumulation
  - Elasticity of the pericardium
- Causes of pericardial tamponade:
  - Pericarditis and malignant invasion of the pericardium
  - Trauma to the heart
  - Diagnostic and therapeutic procedures, e.g., pericardiocentesis, cardiac catheterization, endocardial pacemaker electrodes
  - Rupture of a dissecting aortic aneurysm into the pericardium

Diagnosis

- Signs:
  - Acute development of retrosternal pressure or pain, dyspnea, vertigo, sometimes syncope
- *Findings:*
  1. Clinical triad:
     - Pulsus paradoxus (mandatory): decrease of systolic blood pressure at inspiration by more than 10 mmHg (assessment by blood pressure cuff or intraarterial probe)
     - Elevated venous pressure with Kussmaul's sign: increase in venous pressure on inspiration
     - Diminished arterial blood pressure
       Occasionally:
       a) Broadening of cardiac dullness
       b) Diminished audibility of heart sounds, pericardial rub
       c) Tachycardia
  2. Echocardiography: accumulation of fluid between epicardium and pericardium, so-called "swinging" heart, dorsal deviation of the septum on inspiration, with augmentation of the right and diminution of the left ventricular diameter

Pericardial Tamponade

3. Pericardiocentesis
4. Chest films: spherically contoured heart with short, slender vascular bundle; lungs without pathology (in contrast to left-sided heart failure)
5. ECG (of little value): low voltage; electrical alternation, if present, is suggestive of marked tamponade
6. Right cardiac catheterization: elevated right atrial and right ventricular pressure that increases at each inspiration.

Differential Diagnosis

- Severe congestive heart failure: pulmonary congestion, but no signs of fluid accumulation on echocardiography
- Pulmonary embolism: acute right cardiac strain, pulmonary artery dilated on echocardiography, no pericardial fluid accumulation

Immediate Care

- Pericardiocentesis: the only effective procedure; drainage even of a small volume of fluid can provide relief
- Volume replacement: if pericardiocentesis is not immediately feasible, IV infusion of 500 ml fluid in 10 min, then 100–500 ml/h; if insufficiently effective: dobutamine 2–10 µg/kg/min (drip)

Continuing Care

- Insertion of a pericardial drain
- Surgical intervention if:
  - no fluid can be aspirated;
  - drainage fails to improve the tamponade;
  - trauma is involved.
- Causative treatment:
  - Withdrawal of anticoagulants
  - Corticosteroids, tuberculostatic agents, antibiotics in appropriate cases
  - Intrapericardial application of cytotoxic drugs in case of neoplastic pericarditis

Complications

- Cardiocirculatory arrest
- Rhythm disorders (atrial fibrillation, atrial flutter)
- Late sequela: constrictive pericarditis

Prognosis

Depends on:
- Etiology
- Rapidity of diagnosis and initiation of treatment

Cardiac Arrhythmias

Definition

- The following arrhythmias may give rise to emergencies:
  1. Tachycardia:
     - Paroxysmal supraventricular tachycardia
     - Atrial flutter and fibrillation
     - Ventricular tachycardia
  2. Bradycardia:
     - Complete AV block
     - sick sinus syndrome
  3. Cardiocirculatory arrest:
     - Ventricular fibrillation
     - Asystole
- Circulatory impairment is more likely in the presence of heart disease (coronary heart disease, cardiomyopathy, valvular defects).

Diagnosis

- *Findings:*
  1. Clinical:
     - Tachycardia or bradycardia
     - Regular or irregular heartbeat
  2. ECG: essential for correct diagnosis
  3. Intracorporeal electrogram: usually necessary in conditions involving tachycardia and:
     - Unidentifiable atrial action and/or
     - Wide ventricular complexes
  4. Echocardiography: for detection of atrial activity that is not apparent in surface ECG (subcostal view of right atrium, suprasternal view of left atrium)

Immediate Care

- Refer to discussion of specific forms.
- Hospital referral is usually necessary.

Complications

- In case of persistant rhythm disorders, especially when an organic heart defect is present:
  - Myocardial ischemia
  - Heart failure
  - Arterial hypotension, possibly shock
  - Arterial embolism
  - Cardiocirculatory arrest

Prognosis

- Depends on the nature of the underlying cardiac disorder

Sick Sinus Syndrome

Definition

- Arrhythmias involving a transitory or permanent slowing of sinus rate (to below 50/min)
- Signs:
  - Persistant sinus bradycardia
  - Second-degree sinoatrial (SA) block
  - Bradycardia-tachycardia syndrome
  - Sinus nodal arrest
- Causes: coronary heart disease, sinus node fibrosis

Diagnosis

- *Findings:*
  1. Clinical: Bradycardia (rate below 50/min), which may be constant (in persistent sinus bradycardia) or alternate with phases of normal heart rate (SA block or sinus nodal arrest) or even episodes of tachycardia (bradycardia-tachycardia syndrome)
  2. ECG:
     - Persistent sinus bradycardia, heart rate below 50/min, regular action
     - Second-degree SA block (Mobitz Type I or Wenckebach): progressive shortening of the interval between P waves. The briefest P-P interval is followed by a pause equivalent to less than 2 subsequent P-P intervals.
     - Second-degree SA block, Type II (Mobitz): sudden, unexpected pause lasting twice as long as the previous P-P interval, or some whole multiple thereof
     - Bradycardia-tachycardia syndrome: alternating phases of bradycardia (persistent sinus bradycardia, SA block) with phases of tachycardia (atrial fibrillation, flutter, tachycardia)
     - Sinus nodal arrest: gradually decreasing sinus nodal rate, followed by asystole
  3. Intracorporeal electrogram in conjunction with atrial stimulation: The preautomatic pause following incremental atrial pacing (sinus nodal recovery time) is abnormally prolonged (>1500 ms) in about ¾ of the patients with sick sinus syndrome. Exception: sinus nodal arrest (usually involves normal sinus nodal recovery time)
  4. Holder monitoring ECG: useful for elucidation of sinus nodal arrest, intermittent SA block, and bradycardia-tachycardia syndrome involving only intermittent phases of bradycardia
- *Differential diagnosis:* complete AV block: ECG shows normal P waves not coordinated with the QRS complexes

Immediate Care

- In the event of life-threatening complications (e.g., syncope, vertigo, heart failure), temporary stimulation with isoproterenol or atropine (cf. Complete AV-Nodal Block, p. 88).

Continuing Care

- Pacemaker implantation in case of:
  - Syncope
  - Heart failure
  - Heart rate below 40/min

Complications

- Syncope
- Heart failure
- Embolism (bradycardia-tachycardia syndrome)

Prognosis

- Life expectancy is usually normal.

Complete AV Nodal Block

Definition

- Rhythm disorder characterized by completely interrupted conduction between atrium and ventricle
- Cause: coronary heart disease, fibrosis of the conduction system, (less frequently) digitalis intoxication

Diagnosis

- *Findings:*
  1. Clinical: syncope (in some cases), vertigo, slow heart rate (less than 50/min)
  2. ECG: complete dissociation of atrial and ventricular action; ventricular rate below 50/min, atrial rate considerably faster
- *Differential diagnosis:* sick sinus syndrome: ECG shows atrial rate no faster than ventricular rate

Immediate Care

- If heart rate exceeds 40/min and condition is well tolerated (i.e., patient lacks other symptoms): none
- If heart rate is below 40/min and/or syncope occurs: temporary ventricular pacing. If not feasible: isoproterenol 1–10 µg/min via drip; alternatively: atropine 0.5–1 mg IV

Continuing Care

- Pacemaker implantation in case of permanent complete AV block if any of the following should occur:
  - Syncope
  - Heart failure
  - Heart rate below 40/min

Complications

- Sudden cardiac death
- Heart failure

Prognosis

- Depends on the underlying disorder

Definition

- Usually regular tachycardia of ventricular origin, rate 150–220/min
- Causes: coronary heart disease, cardiomyopathy, QT syndrome, mitral valvular prolapse, myocarditis
- Triggering factors: premature ventricular beats

Diagnosis

- *Findings:*
  1. Clinical: tachycardia, in some cases variable intensity of 1st heart sound (in presence of AV dissociation); rhythm usually regular
  2. ECG: Atrial rate variable, ventricular rate 150–220/min, ventricular complexes broadened; fusion beats and ventricular capture: somewhat irregular ventricular rhythm, ventricular complexes occasionally slender
  3. Intracorporeal electrogram:
     - Atrial and esophageal electrograms: AV dissociation with predominantly negative P waves from the high right atrium, or retrograde conduction; P waves mostly positive in high right atrium
     - His bundle electrogram: absence of H complex preceding the V complex
- *Differential diagnosis:* paroxysmal supraventricular tachycardia and atrial flutter with aberrant conduction:
  - No fusion beats
  - Atrial and esophageal electrograms reveal no AV dissociation; typical flutter waves optional
  - His bundle electrogram: H preceding V, with HV interval 30 ms or longer

Immediate Care

- Lidocaine 50–100 mg IV; may be repeated after 5–10 min. If successful: lidocaine drip, 2–4 mg/min
- If ineffectual, or if complications are present (e.g., heart failure, hypotension, myocardial ischemia): cardioversion (50–400 WS)
- Referral to hospital (in ambulance with continuous monitoring of cardiac rhythm and blood pressure)

Continuing Care

- If tachycardia persists or recurs frequently: programmed right atrial electrical pacing; thereafter (if feasible):
- Switch to oral medication under repeated provocative testing to prevent relapses. Success is likely once electrostimulation fails to elicit ventricular tachycardia.

Complications

- Refer to general section (Cardiac Rhythm Disorders, p. 84), as well as ventricular fibrillation and sudden cardiac death.

Prognosis

- Serious due to likelihood of ventricular fibrillation

Definition

- Sudden outburst of tachycardia in the range of 150–220/min, usually with slender ventricular complexes (0.1 s or less) in ECG
- Cause: WPW (Wolf-Parkinson-White) syndrome, or so-called "longitudinal AV nodal dissociation" (i.e., 2 functionally distinct conduction pathways)
- Precipitating factors: premature beats of supraventricular or ventricular origin; in WPW syndrome, acceleration of the heart rate

Diagnosis

- *Findings:*
  1. Clinical: regular tachycardia, 150–220/min
  2. ECG: same atrial and ventricular rate: 150–220/min; P waves usually hidden in QRS complexes; ventricular complexes usually slender; AV conduction ratio 1:1
  3. Intracorporeal electrogram:
     - Atrial electrogram in the vicinity of the sinus node: atrial waves usually positive, P:QRS ratio 1:1
     - Esophageal electrogram: P:QRS ratio 1:1
     - His bundle electrogram: each V complex preceded by an H complex; HV interval 30 ms or more
- *Differential diagnosis:*
  - Atrial flutter with 2:1 conduction ratio: flutter waves 300/min discernable
  - Ventricular tachycardia: wide ventricular complexes

Immediate Care

- If medication is not available, the diagnosis confirmed, and the patient young: vagal maneuvers (carotid sinus massage, Valsalva's maneuver)
- Otherwise: verapamil 5–10 mg slowly IV (almost always stops the attack)
- If tachycardia persists: referral to hospital

Continuing Care

- If verapamil fails, depending on the patient's condition:
  - Cardioversion in case of hemodynamic impairment, otherwise:
  - Atrial pacing

- If attacks recur frequently, prophylaxis with one or two of the following drugs is indicated: verapamil, beta blockers, cardiac glycosides, quinidine, disopyramide, etc.
  Remember:
  Never combine verapamil with a beta blocker.
- In therapy-resistant cases: His bundle ablation

Complications

- Refer to general section (Cardiac Arrhythmias, p. 84); very rare

Prognosis

- In the absence of organic heart disease, favorable

Definition

- Rhythmic tachycardia (about 300/min) originating in the atrium
- Cause: usually a sequela of organic heart disease (coronary heart disease, carditis, cardiomyopathy)
- Precipitating factor: premature supraventricular beats

Diagnosis

- *Findings:*
  1. Clinical: heartrate 75–300/min; action regular or irregular
  2. ECG: Flutter waves, rate about 300/min; ventricular rate dependent on degree of block; ventricular complexes usually slender
  3. Intracorporeal electrogram:
     - Atrial and esophageal electrograms: atrial waves, about 300/min
     - His bundle electrogram: atrial waves with a rate of approximately 300/min, with HV interval 30 ms or longer
- *Differential diagnosis:*
  - Paroxysmal supraventricular tachycardia: atrial and ventricular frequencies identical, and rate less than 250/min
  - Atrial fibrillation: fibrillation waves with a higher rate (350–600/min) than flutter waves
  - Ventricular tachycardia: wide ventricular complexes

Immediate Care

- If complications arise (e.g., hypotension, heart failure, myocardial ischemia): cardioversion (low energy is usually sufficient: 5–100 Ws)
- If cardioversion is not feasible (due to lack of equipment or success), or no complications present: verapamil 5–10 mg IV, or digoxin 0.5 mg IV to retard the ventricular rate by increasing the degree of AV block
Remember:
In WPW syndrome, start with a class 1A antiarrhythmic drug (see p. 291). If tachycardia continues despite ventricular complexes of normal configuration: verapamil IV

Continuing Care

- If atrial flutter persists, high-frequency atrial stimulation is appropriate. If unsuccessful: cardiac glycosides to reduce ventricular frequency, followed by chemical cardioversion with quinidine (max. 2 g/day); to prevent recurrence: quinidine or disopyramide
- If chemical cardioversion fails: long-term digitalis therapy
- In therapy-resistant cases: ablation of His bundle

Complications

- See general section (Cardiac Arrhythmias, p. 84).

Prognosis

- Depends on the underlying cardiac disorder

Definition

- Irregular tachycardia of atrial origin, rate 350–600/min
- Cause: usually organic heart disease (e.g., coronary heart disease, cardiomyopathy, mitral valve defects); more rarely, hyperthyroidism
- Precipitating factor: supraventricular premature beats

Diagnosis

- *Findings:*
  1. Clinical: heart rate variable, cardiac action irregular
  2. ECG: atrial rate 300–600/min, fibrillation waves; ventricular rate variable, ventricular complexes usually slender
  3. Intracorporeal electrogram:
     - Atrial and esophageal electrogram: fibrillation waves, 300–600/min
     - His bundle electrogram: as above; HV interval 30 ms or longer
- *Differential diagnosis:* atrial flutter: flutter waves uniform and less rapid (300/min)

Immediate Care

- If complications are present (e.g., hypotension, heart failure, myocardial ischemia): cardioversion (100–400 WS)
- If cardioversion is not feasible (lack of equipment or unsuccessful), or complications absent: verapamil 5–10 mg IV or digoxin 0.5 mg IV to slow AV conduction

Remember:

Initial treatment of WPW syndrome should be with a class 1A antiarrhythmic drug (see p. 291), not with verapamil. If ventricular rate still exceeds 100/min after normalization of the QRS complexes, verapamil IV may be added.

Continuing Care

- If atrial fibrillation continues: cardiac glycosides to slow ventricular rate; anticoagulation; thereafter: pharmacologic restoration of sinus rhythm with quinidine (max. 2 g/d)
- Prevention of recurrence: quinidine or disopyramide
- If the latter fail: long-term digitalis therapy, anticoagulation
- In therapy-resistant cases: His-bundle ablation

Complications

- Listed in general section (Cardiac Arrhythmias, p. 84); in addition: systemic embolism, pulmonary embolism

Prognosis

- Depends on the underlying cardiac disorder

Diagnosis

- Typical symptoms: retrosternal pain with or without spread to the left shoulder and left arm lasting for 30 min or more without relief by nitroglycerin
- Less typical symptoms:
  - Upper abdominal pain with sinus bradycardia and/or arterial hypotension (suggestive of inferior infarction)
  - Acute left-sided heart failure
  - Rapid, irregular pulse
- *Findings:*
  1. Clinical: fourth heart sound in uncomplicated infarction; rise in blood pressure possible
  2. Laboratory: increase of the so-called cardiospecific enzymes [CPK (creatine phosphokinase) and CPK-MB (cardiospecific CPK)]
  3. ECG: Tall, peaked T waves, later ST elevation proceeding from the downslope of the R wave
  4. Rhythm surveillance via electronic monitor
  5. PA catheter for assessment of PA pressure and cardiac output for monitoring hemodynamics and control of therapy
- *Differential diagnosis:*
  - Angina pectoris: pain lasts no longer than 20 min, nitrates provide relief; enzymes not enhanced
  - Dissecting aneurysm of the aorta: left-sided pulse often weak, diastolic murmur audible over the base of the heart, no enhancement of enzymes, no signs of infarction in ECG
  - Pericarditis: pericardial rub, usually no enhancement of enzymes; ECG: ST elevation, proceeding from the upstroke of the S wave
  - Pneumothorax: hypersonoric or tympanic resonance of the lungs on percussion; respiration sounds weakened or absent
  - Pulmonary embolism: clinical and electrocardiographic signs of right cardiac strain

Immediate Care

- IV line for infusions
- Pain relief: morphine 3–5 mg IV or meperidine (Demerol) 50 mg IV In case of hypotension: fentanyl 1–5 µg/kg IV

  Sedation: diazepam 5–10 mg IV
- To combat hypotension (usually with bradycardia): atropine 0.5–1 mg IV

Acute Myocardial Infarction

- To treat bradycardia: atropine 0.5–1 mg IV, if:
  - Heart rate is less than 50/min
  - First- or second-degree AV block is present

  If response is inadequate: isoproterenol 1–10 µg/min
- In case of premature beats: lidocaine 50–100 mg IV; may be repeated after 10 min, then continued as IV drip (e.g., 1 g in 500 ml 5% glucose solution at rate of 30 drops/min, equivalent to a dose of 3 mg/min)

  Remember:

  Due to the hazard of potentially fatal disorders of ventricular rhythm, lidocaine is also indicated during transportation to the nearest hospital if the distance is long.
- In case of dyspnea, including incipient pulmonary edema: oxygen, nitroglycerin 0.8–1.6 mg sublingually; for further procedure consult p. 79.
- Cardiocirculatory arrest: see p. 60.

Continuing Care

- In-hospital electrocardiographic monitoring, possibly with hemodynamic surveillance as well (PA catheter)
- Continuation of pain medication (as above), as required
- Heparin drip; if contraindicated, low-dose heparin to prevent clotting
- Nitrate in low-dosed drip as routine precaution in every case of infarction efficacy as yet unproved!)
- In shock, treatment must be adjusted in accordance with the hemodynamic situation (refer to p. 69).
- In acute pulmonary edema (refer to p. 79).
- In heart failure: higher-dosed infusion of nitrate, diuretics (e.g., furosemide 20–40 mg IV), dobutamine drip 2–10 µg/kg/min, cardiac glycosides (e.g., digoxin 0.25–0.5 mg IV)
- In arterial hypotension:
  - If heart rate is less than 60/min: atropine 0.5–1 mg IV.
  - If filling pressure is less than 12 mmHg: volume replacement with simultaneous hemodynamic monitoring (see p. 70).
- In cardiogenic shock (refer to p. 69).
- In case of arterial hypertension in excess of 200/110 mmHg: nifedipine 10–20 mg orally, or other antihypertensive drugs
- Systemic or intracoronary thrombolysis
- Rhythm disorders:

  a) Supraventricular premature beats: no therapy required

  b) Hemodynamically relevant ventricular premature beats: lidocaine

c) Ventricular tachycardia: lidocaine 50–100 mg IV; if ineffectual: cardioversion

d) Ventricular fibrillation: See Cardiac Arrest, p. 60.

e) Atrial fibrillation or flutter: verapamil 5–10 mg IV; cardiac glycosides may also be appropriate. If ventricular rate fails to decelerate or the patient is in critical condition: cardioversion

f) Sinus bradycardia: atropine 0.5–1 mg IV, provided:
   - Heart rate is below 50/min; no premature ventricular beats
   - Heart rate is below 60/min with premature ventricular beats
   If ineffective: Isoproterenol

g) AV block:
   - 1st degree: no treatment required
   - 2nd degree: QRS duration 0.1 s or less, and heart rate 50/min or more: no treatment required. QRS duration 0.1 s and heart rate below 50/min: atropine 0.5–1 mg IV. If ineffective: temporary ventricular pacing. QRS duration more than 0.1 s: treatment as above
   - 3rd degree: Temporary ventricular pacing

h) Bundle branch block: temporary pacemaker in case of:
   - Recent right bundle branch block with left anterior hemiblock or left posterior hemiblock
   - Recent bundle branch block with 1st degree AV block
   - Alternating blockade of right and left bundle branches

i) Asystole: See Cardiac Arrest, p. 60.

Complications

- Hemodynamic disorders: congestive heart failure, cardiogenic shock (about 15%)
- Rhythm disorders:
  - Premature beats (supraventricular, ventricular)
  - Atrial fibrillation, atrial flutter
  - Ventricular tachycardia
  - Ventricular fibrillation (about 8%)
  - AV block
  - Bundle branch and branch blocks
- Mechanical disorders:
  - Septal rupture
  - Free wall rupture
  - Rupture of papillary muscle
- Pericarditis
- Thromboembolism:
  - Venous: potential source of pulmonary embolism
  - Intraventricular: potential source of systemic arterial embolism

Unstable Angina Pectoris

Definition

- Angina pectoris is referred to as unstable in case of:
  - sudden onset without prior symptoms;
  - abrupt increase in frequency, duration, and intensity of pain in stable angina pectoris;
  - occurrence of attacks of pain at rest or at night.

Pathophysiology

- Aside from organic stenosis, other factors are probably involved, e.g., spasms of the coronary arteries, and probably reversible platelet deposits.

Diagnosis

- 1. Clinical: See Definition.
  2. ECG: ST depression or elevation during pain attack that fails to resolve immediately thereafter
  3. Exercise ECG: can be carried out only at lowest exercise level (25–50 W)
  4. Laboratory: no enzyme enhancement
  5. Coronary angiography: indicated if medical therapy fails, or after disappearance of acute symptoms

Differential Diagnosis

- Myocardial infarction: lengthy persistance of pain and failure to respond to nitroglycerin; enzyme enhancement, typical ECG alterations

Therapy

- Initially, conservative medical treatment to stabilize the patient; a combination of 3 drugs usually required
- Nitroglycerin drip 2–6 mg/h (if necessary up to 10 mg/h)
- Calcium entry blockers:
  - Nifedipine orally (20 mg q 2 h, max. dosage 160 mg/day) or as IV infusion (5 mg in 4–8 h)
  - Verapamil orally (80 mg q 3 h, max. dosage 800 mg/day) or as infusion (0.1 mg/kg/h initially, max. dosage 1.5 mg/kg/d)
  - Diltiazem orally (60–120 mg t.i.d.)
- Beta blockers orally (e.g., metoprolol 50–100 mg b.i.d. or atenolol 50–100 mg once a day)
- Heparin: infusion of therapeutic dosage

- If the response is inadequate ($\frac{1}{4}$–$\frac{1}{3}$ of all cases): Coronary arteriography is indicated. Thereafter, depending on the findings, coronary balloon dilation or aortocoronary bypass surgery may be appropriate.

Complications

- Sudden cardiac death in 5–10%
- Myocardial infarction in about 15%

Prognosis

- Serious because of potential complications. About $\frac{2}{3}$–$\frac{3}{4}$ of the patients can be converted to a stable form; in such cases, coronary arteriography should be performed in a symptomless phase.

Dissecting Aortic Aneurysm

Definition

- Splitting of the tunica media by a dissecting layer of blood emanating from intramural hemorrhage
- Stanford classification:
  Type A (⅔ of cases): involvement of ascending aorta
  Type B (⅓ of cases): ascending aorta not involved
- Cause: media necrosis
  Predisposing conditions: arterial hypertension, Marfan's syndrome, aortic valvular disease

Diagnosis

- Presenting symptoms:
  Severe thoracic pain of abrupt onset, collapse or shock
- *Findings:*
  1. Clinical signs depend on the site of the dissection and are thus variable:
     - Aortic valvular incompetence
     - Blood pressure difference between upper and lower extremities or between left and right upper arms
     - Pulsations at the sternoclavicular joint
  2. Laboratory (hematology): in some cases, drop in Hb and Hct, indicating bleeding
  3. ECG: No signs of infarction (important in differential diagnosis)
  4. Chest x-ray: occasionally, typical signs, e.g., circumscribed dilation of the aorta, doubly contoured aortic wall, aortic walls no longer parallel; pleural effusions (hematothorax) or broadened heart shadow (hematopericardium) less common
  5. Echocardiography: doubly contoured aortic wall; occasionally, evidence of aortic regurgitation, pericardial effusions, pleural effusions; transesophageal view essential to determine extent
  6. CT scan: intima avulsion, visualization of lumens, displaced intima calcifications, dilation of aorta, pericardial effusions; also suitable for course monitoring
  7. Supravalvular aortography: most reliable method of diagnosis and localization
- *Differential diagnosis:*
  - Myocardial infarction: absence of pulse differences; enzyme enhancement, typical ECG changes
  - Acute pericarditis: pulse differences absent, no aortic valvular incompetence, typical pericardial rub
  - Pneumothorax: hypersonoric or tympanic resonance on percussion; respiration sounds on auscultation of the lungs weak or absent
  - Pulmonary embolism: clinical and electrocardiographic signs of right heart strain

Immediate Care

- Absolute bedrest
- Analgesia: morphine 5–10 mg IV
- In case of hypovolemia: volume replacement

Continuing Care

- 1. Early surgical intervention desirable in type A aneurysm
     Contraindications:
     - Concurrent disorders with unfavorable prognosis
     - Irreversible infarction (cardiac, cerebral, renal, etc.)
     In type B aneurysms, surgical intervention depends on occurrence of complications:
     - Progression of dissection
     - Hemorrhage
     - Uncontrollable hypertension
     - Ischemia of other organs
     - Saccular aneurysm
  2. Medical therapy with antihypertensive drugs in type B aneurysm, or in type A aneurysm in which surgery is contraindicated
     - In hypertension, initial treatment consists of: methyldopa (250–500 mg IV) or clonidine (0.15–0.3 mg IV); sodium nitroprusside (0.5–8 µg/kg/min drip) may be substituted.
     - If blood pressure is normal: reserpine and/or propranolol
     - In hypotension (systolic pressure below 120 mmHg): Plasma expanders

Complications

- Rupture of the aneurysm into the pericardium
- Cardiogenic shock consequent upon aortic valvular incompetence or myocardial infarction
- Rupture of the aneurysm into the pleural or peritoneal cavity, or the retroperitoneum
- Organ ischemia due to compression of departing vessels

Prognosis

- Serious; better in type B than in type A
- Lethality in medically-treated type A aneuryms about 65%, in type B aneurysm about 25%

Pulmonary Embolism

Definition

- Acute partial obstruction of the pulmonary circulation by embolic particles, leading to secondary arterial spasms and pulmonary hypertension with right-sided heart failure; followed by pulmonary infarction within 12–72 h in about 40% of cases

Etiology

- Usually (in 90% of cases) thrombosis of pelvic or deep leg veins, more rarely thrombi originating in the right atrium (in atrial fibrillation) or the right ventricle (in right-sided endocarditis)
- *Predisposing factors:*
  Age, immobilization, recent surgery, heart failure, pregnancy, oral contraceptives, malignant disease, overweight

Diagnosis

- *Symptoms:*
  - Sudden dyspnea and palpitations
  - Thoracic pain, vertigo, (occasionally) syncope
  - Hypotension, clinical evidence of shock
  - In pulmonary infarction: hemoptysis, pleural pain
- *Findings:*
  1. Clinical:
     - Cyanosis, tachycardia, dyspnea
     - Distended cervical veins
     - Right ventricular pulsations enhanced
     - Abnormal splitting of the 2nd heart sound with emphasis on the pulmonic 2nd component; 3rd and 4th heart sounds occasionally audible below the right substernal margin
     - Lungs: pleural rub possibly accompanying pulmonary infarction
  2. ECG: acute right cardiac strain (P in II, III, and aVF $>0.25\,\text{mV}$, and in V_1 and $V_2 >0.15\,\text{mV}$
     Dextroanterior rotation of QRS axis: S_1–Q_3 type
     Acute right ventricular strain: high R waves with negative T waves in V_1–V_4
  3. Chest x-ray: prominence of the pulmonary artery, and lack of vascular shadows in the periphery; the heart may appear enlarged. In pulmonary infarction, opacity of individual lung fields may be present.
  4. Pulmonary radioisotope perfusion scan: circumscribed perfusion defect. If findings are normal, hemodynamically significant pulmonary embolization is unlikely.

5. Hemodynamics: Central venous pressure may exceed 20 cm H_2O in severe pulmonary embolism. Pulmonary arterial pressure is elevated (mean >25 mmHg); wedge pressure is normal.
6. Pulmonary arteriography (most accurate method): filling defects or abrupt cutoff of a pulmonary arterial segment
   Remember:
   The pulmonary artery catheter should be introduced via an arm vein rather than a femoral vein to avoid new emboli.
7. Echocardiography: suprasternal dilation of the pulmonary artery; precordial or subxiphoidal view: dilation of the right ventricle, paradoxical excursions of the septum, normal size of left ventricle
8. Blood gas analysis: arterial pO_2 usually less than 80 mmHg, pCO_2 variable (usually below 40 mmHg)

- *Differential diagnosis:*
  - Pneumothorax: hypersonoric resonance; respiration sounds weakened or absent
  - Myocardial infarction: lack of right cardiac failure, typical changes in ECG, CK elevation
  - Dissecting aortic aneurysm: aortic valvular incompetence, circumscribed dilation of the aorta on x-ray, doubly contoured aortic wall on echocardiography
  - Pericarditis: pericardial rub, no evidence of right heart strain, ECG changes typical of pericarditis

Immediate Care

- Elevation of head and thorax
- Oxygen via mask 10 L/min
- Establishment of IV access route
- Analgesia: opiates (morphine 5–10 mg IV)
- Sedation: diazepam 5–10 mg IV

Continuing Care

- Small vessel emboli: bedrest (about 7 days), heparin; later, coumadin derivatives
- Major pulmonary embolism with signs of right ventricular strain: fibrinolysis, followed by heparin and coumadin derivatives
  Alternatively: local thrombolysis with streptokinase via pulmonary artery catheter
- Cardiogenic shock (or if fibrinolysis should be contraindicated or ineffectual): insertion of a Greenfield catheter, or thoracotomy for embolectomy, followed by heparin and coumadin derivatives

- Prevention of recurrence:
  1. Coumadin derivatives for 6–9 months, or
  2. Implantation of caval filter if:
     - anticoagulants for prevention are contraindicated;
     - embolism recurs in spite of proper anticoagulation;
     - pulmonary hypertension develops as a sequela to chronically recurrent pulmonary embolism and nonpreventable phlebothrombosis;
     - acute calf vein thrombosis develops with large, free-floating thrombi without possibility of thrombolysis or thrombectomy.
  3. Venous thrombectomy in event of recent pelvic venous thrombosis with free-floating thrombi

Complications

- Cardiocirculatory arrest
- Cardiogenic shock
- Chronic pulmonary hypertension due to recurrent embolism
- Infection of pulmonary infarction: infarction pneumonia; abscess formation

Prognosis

- Short-term prognosis: serious (sudden death in 20–40% of cases)
- Long-term prognosis: favorable, provided:
  - pulmonary hypertension does not develop following the acute phase, and prevention of recurrence is effective (recurrence to be expected in 30–50% of cases);
  - predisposing factors can be influenced.

Hypertensive Crisis and Hypertensive Emergencies

Definition

- Sudden rise in blood pressure with consequent impairment of central nervous system, cardiac, or renal function

Diagnosis

- Symptoms:
  - Hypertensive encephalopathy with headache, nausea, vomiting, spots before the eyes, muscular palsy, aphasia, scotoma (possibly, amaurosis), epileptiform seizures, apathy, somnolence, coma
  - Cardiac symptoms: angina pectoris, resting dyspnea, pulmonary edema, myocardial infarction
  - Ocular symptoms: impairment of vision, papillary edema, retinal bleeding
  - Impairment of renal function with oliguria
- Cause: hypertension of any cardiovascular origin
- *Findings:*
  1. Clinical: Blood pressure 200/120 mmHg or higher; neurological status
  2. Laboratory: BUN augmented in some cases
  3. Fundoscopy: grade 4 retinopathy
  4. ECG: signs of left ventricular hypertrophy usually present; however, ECG may appear normal.
- *Differential diagnosis:*
  - Stroke, acute hyperthyroidism; sudden increase of blood pressure lacking in both

Immediate Care

- Furosemide 20–40 mg IV
- Antihypertensive drugs:
  - Nifedipine 20 mg sublingually; may be repeated after 5–20 min if necessary
  - Hydralazine 12.5 mg IV or IM (intramuscular); if no effect after another 30 min, 25 mg IV or IM
  - If the above measures fail: diazoxide 75–300 mg rapidly (within less than 30 s) IV or
  - Sodium nitroprusside drip, starting with 20 µg/min, up to maximum of 0.5–8 µg/kg/min

- In pheochromocytoma: phentolamine 5 mg IV
  Remember:
  The therapeutic goal in the first few days is reduction of blood pressure to levels around 140/100 mmHg. Do not allow blood pressure to drop below 170/100 mmHg in hypertensive crises with malignant hypertension and hypertensive encephalopathy with fundal pathology (hazard of blindness due to deficient autoregulation of the retinal arteries).

Complications

- Acute pulmonary edema
- Cerebral hemorrhage
- Dissecting aortic aneurysm
- Acute myocardial infarction

Prognosis

- Favorable, provided diagnosis is made promptly and treatment initiated immediately. Depends on the following:
  - Extent of rise in blood pressure
  - Baseline blood pressure
  - Duration of hypertension history (and thus extent of vascular damage)
  - Underlying disorder
  - Frequency of recurrence

Adult Respiratory Distress Syndrome (ARDS)

Definition

- Adult respiratory distress syndrome (ARDS), synonymous with acute respiratory failure
  This syndrome is not an etiologically defined disease entity; it refers to a similar reaction of initially intact lungs to any of several pulmonary and extrapulmonary disorders.
  1. Clinical symptoms and morphologic changes are uniform and typical of ARDS as follows:
     - Acute respiratory failure at onset
     - Disseminated interstitial pulmonary changes
     - Progressive respiratory failure in the further course
  2. Morphologically, ARDS initially involves diffuse impairment of pulmonary capillary permeability, with loss of plasma and cellular components into the interstitial spaces.
  3. ARDS is always a secondary disease with a typical, but highly variable course. The course is also influenced by the underlying disorder and its peculiar dynamics, as well as by further complications.
  Remember:
  Not all cases of acute respiratory failure with radiographic signs of interstitial pulmonary changes are due to ARDS. There are several pulmonary diseases of exogenous or endogenous origin that are similar in appearance, but have a different pathogenesis, and do not involve capillary damage.

Etiology – Pathogenesis

- Damage to pulmonary capillaries with effusion and subsequent proliferation as well as damage to alveolar epithelium and interference with surfactant function are the basic mechanisms in pathogenesis of ARDS.

Adult Respiratory Distress Syndrome (ARDS)

- The etiology may involve any of several disorders compiled in the Task Force Report of the US National Heart and Lung Institute, some of which are listed here:
  - Circulatory shock, regardless of origin
  - Septicemia
  - Polytrauma
  - Consumption coagulopathy (= disseminated intravascular coagulation)
  - Fat embolism
  - Aspiration
  - Burns
  - Inhalation of toxic fumes
  - Acute pancreatitis
  - Acute renal failure
  - Massive transfusion
  - Viral pneumonia
  - Acute oral intoxication

Diagnosis – Differential Diagnosis

- The classic symptomatology of ARDS can develop within hours, or after a latency period of several days, depending on the intensity of the precipitating cause. This underlines the necessity of frequent monitoring of patients exposed to known potential causes of ARDS.
- Clinical symptoms are usually dominated by signs of acute respiratory failure:
  - Tachypnea and dyspnea with labored respiration
  - Pallor and flaring of nostrils
  - Signs of circulatory centralization
  - Notably weak cough
  - On auscultation and percussion no typical findings except for occasional wheezing, i.e., marked discrepancy to other clinical evidence
- Blood gases:
  - $P_{aO_2} < 60$ mmHg, increasing somewhat when O_2 concentration of inspired air is increased
  - P_{aCO_2} initially < 40 mmHg, indicating enhancement of ventilation as a compensatory mechanism ($pH_a > 7.4$); with increasing fatigue as the course progresses, $P_{aCO_2} > 40$ mmHg ($pH_a < 7.4$)
- *Tracheal aspirates:*
  Quantitatively and qualitatively usually normal or viscid

- *Chest x-ray:*
  - Marked initial discrepancy between clinical symptoms and unremarkable radiologic findings
  - Diffuse opacities initially in some cases
  - Typical radiologic changes: finely to coarsely spotted, striated, or reticular disseminated infiltrations, usually symmetrical, and positive air bronchograms; heart usually of normal size; in full-blown ARDS, opacity of entire lung
- *Mechanics of respiration and gas exchange:*
  - Functional residual capacity diminished
  - Compliance reduced
  - Vital capacity diminished
  - Increased right-to-left shunt during inhalation of pure O_2
  - Increased difference between alveolar and arterial O_2 partial pressure ($A\text{-}aD_{O_2}$) and between inspiratory and arterial O_2 partial pressure ($i\text{-}aD_{O_2}$)
  - Increased dead space ratio (V_D/V_T)
- *Hemodynamic changes:*
  - Normal CVP
  - Cardiac output normal or increased at first, lessening later
  - Pulmonary vascular resistance elevated
  - Pulmonary capillary wedge pressure lowered
- *Differential diagnosis:*
  - Pulmonary edema of cardiac origin
  - Hypervolemia (fluid lung)
  - Bacterial bronchopneumonia
  - Allergic alveolitis
  - Goodpasture's syndrome
  - Pulmonary involvement in so-called inflammatory systemic or inflammatory rheumatic diseases (e.g., SLE [systemic lupus erythematosus], rheumatoid arthritis)

Continuing Care

- Centers on prompt initiation of volume-regulated ventilation with PEEP
- Precise balancing and cautious replacement of fluids
- Large doses of methylprednisolone (2 g q 6 h IV for 48 h); possibly effective only in early stages
- Heparin in low dosages; in case of threatened or manifest disseminated intravascular coagulation, therapeutic dosage required
- Concurrent treatment of the underlying disorder
- Early initiation of hemodialysis or hemofiltration in appropriate cases

Adult Respiratory Distress Syndrome (ARDS)

Complications

- Secondary bacterial infection
- Pulmonary hypertension and right cardiac failure in case ARDS progresses
- Acute renal failure
- Additional alveolar damage by barotrauma due to necessity of high-pressure ventilation and toxic concentrations of O_2

Prognosis

- Lethal outcome in 60–80% of cases, depending on underlying disorder and adequacy of treatment
- Improvement of prognosis by early initiation of vigorous therapy, especially mechanical ventilation
- Complete recovery possible, even from advanced ARDS in individual cases

Definition

- The term aspiration syndrome (Mendelson's syndrome, aspiration pneumonia) refers to the pulmonary reaction to diffuse aspiration of acidic gastric juice. It involves typical clinical symptoms and progressive morphologic changes of lung parenchyma as in ARDS.
  - The pH of the gastric juice is of critical importance. pH below 2.5 is associated with severe symptoms.
  - Secondary superinfection is a potential hazard, but not in early stages.
  - Symptoms are closely related to those produced by toxic damage consequent upon inhalation of noxious gases.
- Mendelson's classical aspiration syndrome must be differentiated from aspiration of large amounts of blood, undigested gastric contents, or foreign bodies that lead to atelectasis by occluding large bronchi. Tracheal blockage may affect the entire airways system; the extreme form is reflexive asphyxia due to an alimentary bolus in a major bronchus.

  In this context, secondary bacterial infections in completely or partially occluded, poorly ventilated segments become highly relevant, and may give rise to aspiration pneumonia or pulmonary abscesses.
- Aspiration may be complicated if the stomach contains substances directly toxic to the lungs, e.g., after oral intake of alkylated phosphates or paraquat.

Etiology

- Inability of the patient to guide the contents of the laryngopharynx, especially in neurologic disorders
- Deficient cough and gagging reflexes in comatose patients, especially in case of poisoning
- Regurgitation due to deficient gastric muscle tone
- Inadequate blockage of endotracheal tube or incomplete gastric drainage (clamped-off gastric tube in presence of overfilled stomach)
- Esophageotracheal fistulas

Diagnosis

- Diagnosis may be difficult if the aspiration event is not witnessed.
- Clinical symptoms develop after a variable latent period:
  - The larger the quantity and the lower the pH, the more severe the reaction.

- Clinical symptoms:
  - Cyanosis
  - Tachycardia, dyspnea, tachypnea
  - Moist and dry rales
  - Hypotension
  - Tracheobronchorrhea
  - Pulmonary edema due to exudation

  Remember:
  The widespread exudation and tracheal and bronchial secretion at onset may lead to confusion with pulmonary edema of cardiac origin.

- Blood gas analysis:
  - Hypoxemia, initial hypocapnia; hypercapnia as lung damage progresses
  - Acidosis of variable degree

- Clinical and blood gas changes due to aspiration of blood and undigested gastric contents are minimal at first in comatose patients and those with impaired consciousness, so that the diagnosis cannot be established until atelectasis and aspiration pneumonia develop. An early clue is provided by mechanical suction of gastric contents from the bronchial system. Physical signs depend on the extent and position of the occlusion, and on which part of the lungs has collapsed.

- *Chest x-ray:*
  - Mendelson's syndrome:
    Diffuse alveolar congestion over *both* lungs
    Interstitial pulmonary edema
  - Massive aspiration:
    Atelectasis and signs of diminished ventilation
    Aspiration pneumonia in poorly ventilated parts of the lung
    Asymmetrical findings
    Remember:
    Radiologic signs may be absent at first, but chest x-ray is always indicated for purposes of later comparison. The superior segment of the right or left lower lobes is often affected in bedridden patients.

- *Differential diagnosis:*
  - Pulmonary edema due to other causes
  - Atelectasis due to a plug of bronchial mucous
  - Lobar pneumonia

Immediate Care

- Bronchial toilet and clearing of foreign matter from blocked airways in case of massive aspiration:
  - Endotracheal intubation
  - Endotracheal suction
  - Vibratory massage
  - Chest physiotherapy
  - Position conducive to drainage
  - Bronchoscopy if these measures fail to bring about significant improvement
  - Bronchial lavage with physiologic saline to loosen encrusted secretions; additives produce no improvement
  Remember:
  In classic Mendelson's syndrome, bronchoscopy is necessary neither for diagnosis nor therapy.

Continuing Care

- Prompt initiation of PEEP ventilation
- Basic intensive care with input-output balancing and monitoring
- Steroids useful only if given within 20 min after aspiration; controversial, because they increase susceptibility to bacterial infection
- Prophylactic use of antibiotics contraindicated
- Heparinization

Complications

- Secondary colonization by microorganisms consequent upon massive aspiration
- ARDS in the later course of diffuse aspiration of gastric juice

Prognosis

- Depends on how early diagnosis is established, and emergency treatment *and* PEEP ventilation are initiated

Definition

- Pneumonias requiring intensive care may be classified as follows:
  1. *Primary pneumonia* contracted outside the hospital, caused by the following pathogens:
     - Viral or mycoplasmal organisms
     - Pneumococcus spp.
     - Haemophilus influenzae
     - Klebsiella spp.
     - Staphylococcus aureus
       Severe courses necessitating mechanical ventilation are rare.
  2. *Primary atypical pneumonia* caused by viral and mycoplasmal agents: The clinical course is more severe than that of classic bacterial pneumonia, and a particularly fulminant form may develop involving:
     - Rapid progression of acute respiratory failure and ARDS
     - Cardiocirculatory shock
     - Acute renal failure
     - Disseminated intravascular coagulation
     - Hepatic damage
     Legionnaire's pneumonia is in this category.
  3. *Secondary pneumonia* is contracted in the hospital. Immunodeficient ICU patients are susceptible, and it is often consequent upon aspiration, deficient hygiene in patients on mechanical ventilation, and uncritical employment of antibiotics. Aspiration of pathogens is apparently the most important factor in colonization of the respiratory tract and development of pneumonia. Microorganisms from the oropharynx or even from the stomach may enter the lungs, leading to development of overt pneumonia in immunocompromised individuals.
     The most important causative agents are:
     - Gram-negative bacteria
     - Staphylococci
     - Facultative pathogens

Diagnosis

- Diagnosis of primary pneumonia is based on clinical and x-ray findings and identification of the pathogen.
  Noteworthy features of primary atypical pneumonia include:
  - Onset with nonspecific signs of a "cold" with fever and dry cough
  - In severe cases, history often revealing unusual strain and factors that weaken resistance
  - Discrepancy between radiographic findings (focal to widespread opacities) and scanty physical pathology
  - Lack of demonstrable pathogens in tracheal secretions

● Secondary pneumonia acquired in the hospital may be difficult to diagnose, since there may be many causes of fever and auscultation findings, and radiologic findings may not be clearly identifiable as pneumonic infiltrations. Besides, identification of pathogens in and of itself does afford proof of a clinically relevant infection. Since there are no specific criteria, so-called "sensitive criteria" are used:
  – Serial radiographic findings
  – Auscultation findings
  – Temperature
  – WBC
  – Serial bacteriology with quantitation
  Diagnosis of secondary pneumonia is based on the totality of findings and course.

● *Differential diagnosis:*
  – Pulmonary infarction
  – Pulmonary edema of cardiac origin
  – Aspiration
  – ARDS
  – Immunologic and autoimmunologic events in the lungs

Intensive Care

● Bacterial pneumonia:
  – Antimicrobial therapy must be consistent with established rules of antibiotic treatment.
  – Whether mechanical ventilation is indicated depends on the extent to which oxygenation is diminished and CO_2 is retained (for guidelines, see p. 264). The indication is given if signs of development of ARDS are present.
  – In *primary* bacterial pneumonia there is an enhanced risk of secondary pulmonary contamination by resistant microorganisms, so that the decision in favor of mechanical ventilation must be based on stringent criteria. It depends on whether adequate P_{aO_2} can be maintained by O_2 insufflation, on the patient's overall strength, and on whether *active* lung care (expectoration, breathing exercises, vibratory massage, chest physiotherapy, vapor inhalation) is feasible (cooperation by the patient, tolerance of physiotherapy)
  – The decision in favor of mechanical ventilation is easier in elderly and/or weakened patients in whom pneumonia poses a vital hazard to cardiocirculatory function, or if pneumonia has led to other extrapulmonary complications or metabolic decompensation (e.g., diabetic coma triggered by massive bacterial pneumonial infection).

- Primary atypical pneumonias with severe course:
  - Mechanical ventilation should be instituted promptly, using PEEP right from the start.
    It is also indicated in the event of disseminated intravascular coagulation and/or acute renal failure, even if the usual criteria of respiratory function seem to indicate the potential for compensation.
  - Immediate IV heparinization in therapeutic dosages
  - Early initiation of hemodialysis (see guidelines p. 311).
  - Generous administration of steroids as in ARDS (p. 111).
  - Tetracyclines, since mycoplasma infection cannot be ruled out in initial differential diagnosis
    Remember:
    Frequent blood gas analyses and systematic intensive care and monitoring are required, since the patient's condition may deteriorate within a few hours.

Prognosis

- Fulminant atypical pneumonias with acute respiratory failure and transition to ARDS has the worst prognosis. Prompt initiation of mechanical ventilation seems to be successful in individual cases.

Acquired Immune Deficiency Syndrome (AIDS)

Definition

- Acquired immune deficiency caused by a virus. New nomenclature: HIV (human immunodeficiency virus); also has been referred to as HTLV-3 (human T-cell leukemia virus type 3)

Etiology

- The virus is found in blood, saliva, and semen. It is transmitted mainly by sexual contact, blood transfusions, and blood-to-blood contact.

Diagnosis

- Serological testing (evidence of antibodies by enzyme-linked immunosorbent assay [ELISA], etc.)
- Immunological deviations typical of AIDS:
  1. Lymphopenia
  2. T_4-lymphocyte deficiency; altered T_4/T_8 ratio
- Hyperactive B cells
- Anergia
- Polyclonal enhancement mainly of IgG (immunoglobulin G) and IgA (immunoglobulin A)
- Clinical picture in overt stage:
  Dominated by opportunistic infections or typical neoplasms:
  1. Kaposi's sarcoma
  2. Lymphomas of the CNS
  Opportunistic infections:
  1. Pneumonia, encephalitis, meningitis, caused by:
     a) Pneumocystis
     b) Toxoplasma
     c) Cytomegalovirus
  2. Candida infection
  3. Disseminated atypical mycobacteriosis
  4. Disseminated histoplasmosis

Differential Diagnosis

- Immunosuppression caused by other factors, especially cytotoxic or other medication
  Malignomas of any type

Therapy

- No causative therapy available to date
- Specific treatment of opportunistic infections
  Important! Psychosocial and nursing care of AIDS patients are the most important aspects.

Definition

- *Chronic bronchopulmonary disorders* involve episodes of acute respiratory failure occurring with increasing frequency during a course of many years as global respiratory insufficiency increases and cor pulmonale develops. Intensive therapy, especially mechanical ventilation, is aimed at tiding the patient over such events, and overcoming complications and infections that may have elicited them in the first place. In terminal stages, it is not reasonable to place patients on mechanical ventilation if they are not likely ever to become weaned from it again.

- Acute exacerbation of the chronic obstructive bronchopulmonary syndrome involves an additional acute increase of pressure in the pulmonary circulation and strain on the right heart. Combined with global respiratory failure, this may give rise to acute cardiac decompensation. In such cases, improvement of blood gas levels usually suffices to bring about cardiac recovery.

- In *bronchial asthma,* severe, protracted attacks (status asthmaticus) may necessitate intensive therapy with mechanical ventilation.

Pathogenesis

- Airway constriction always involves 3 basic mechanisms, which participate to varying extents and must be considered in therapy:
  1. Increased smooth muscle tone in the bronchial wall (bronchial spasms)
  2. Increased secretion of tenacious mucous (hypersecretion, dyskinesia)
  3. Inflammatory swelling of the bronchial mucosa (mucosal edema)

- Initially, bronchial spasms usually predominate. As the condition persists longer, the accumulation of tenacious mucous gains in importance.

- Younger patients with bronchial asthma tend to be initially afflicted by bronchial spasms. In older patients with chronic obstructive bronchitis, retention of mucous tends to predominate right from the start.

Diagnosis

- Two types of patients with different prognoses and thus with different indications for intensive care may be distinguished:
  1. Patients with less obvious symptoms of bronchitis, in whom emphysema is the predominant disorder: once conservative measures have been exhausted and terminal overall respiratory failure has set in, the prognosis in such patients is very poor, and mechanical ventilation is no longer indicated.

Acute Bronchial Obstruction

2. Patients in whom symptoms of bronchitis and bronchial obstruction predominate, and who develop signs of impaired gas exchange, pulmonary artery hypertension, and right-sided heart failure fairly early in the course: Acute decompensation in such patients responds better to therapy. Generous use of mechanical ventilation appears justified, since recompensation is feasible. Still, the prospects for overcoming acute decompensation in these cases decrease as concomitant cor pulmonale progresses.

- The most important functional parameter in assessment of the course is peak flow, which can be easily and repeatedly determined in an in-hospital setting.

Immediate Care

- Beta-2 sympathomimetic drugs in metered aerosol canisters to be administered by a physician (patient unlikely to use them correctly in status arthmaticus)
- Theophylline IV (e.g., 6 mg/kg slowly IV, followed by 240 mg/2–4 h as a continuous drip); plasma theophylline levels to be monitored if feasible
- If ineffectual: terbutaline 0.25–0.5 mg s.c.
- Corticosteroids (e.g., 100–250 mg prednisolone IV), should severe bronchial obstruction persist

Continuing Care

- Before a decision in favor of mechanical ventilation is made, all available conservative measures for treating *obstructive lung disease,* including use of O_2, must be attempted. Patients with severe pneumonia as the main cause of acute respiratory failure are the only exception to this rule.
  - Continued systemic administration of broncholytic drugs. Theophylline also exerts a positive inotropic effect on the diaphragm muscle; dosage control by assay of plasma levels
  - Secretomotory drugs IV (significant effect not proven)
  - Aerosol therapy with spray or ultrasonic nebulizers (bronchial dilating agents, secretomotory agents)
  - Physiotherapy, including postural drainage, breathing exercises, and possibly translaryngeal endobronchial suction
  - Continuous O_2 insufflation
  - Corticosteroids in case of severe, persistent, acute bronchial obstruction
  - Systemic antibiotics in case of purulent sputum or evidence of pulmonary infiltration

- Therapeutic options in *concomitant cor pulmonale:*
  - Digitalization (caution: sensitivity to digitalis is enhanced in cor pulmonale)
  - Diuretics: Hematocrit must be monitored; phlebotomy indicated if hematocrit exceeds 55–60 vol.%
  - Heparin to prevent thromboembolic complications
  - Nitrates for acute reduction of pulmonary artery pressure
- Mechanical ventilation with intermittent positive pressure via mouthpiece (IPPB = intermittent positive pressure breathing), which can be carried out only with the patient's cooperation, occupies an intermediate position. Restlessness, tachypnea, and dyspnea often result in counterbreathing, causing the patient to tire rapidly.
  Remember:
  Never force IPPB on an unwilling patient.
- Indications for mechanical ventilation:
  The generally accepted criteria for decision in favor of mechanical ventilation in patients with nonobstructive acute respiratory failure do not apply automatically to patients with obstructive respiratory failure. Clinical factors are of prime importance; serial assessment of blood gases is essential, since these chronically ill patients have a number of adaptative mechanisms enabling them to tolerate even markedly pathological deviations fairly well, and rendering interpretation of one-time data difficult. The most relevant criteria are:
1. Clinical signs:
   - Severe dyspnea
   - Depressed respiration (slow, superficial breathing)
   - Cyanosis despite administration of O_2
   - Increasing exhaustion and inability to expectorate by coughing
   - Increasing confusion or clouding of consciousness
   - Cardiac rhythm disorders
   - Hypotension
2. Blood gas levels:
   - P_{aO_2} < 40–50 mmHg
   - P_{aCO_2} > 70–80 mmHg
   - pH_a < 7.2–7.3
3. Development of a hypoventilation-hypercapnia syndrome with hazard of CO_2 narcosis despite correct O_2 insufflation

Acute Bronchial Obstruction

- Ventilating apparatus:
  1. In acute bronchial obstruction, pressure-limited units with variable flow are best (see p. 266). They should be equipped with nebulizers for medication and be adjustable to provide large tidal volume at low flow (low-flow principle). Assisted ventilation is preferable. These patients must be very carefully monitored.
  2. In acute bronchial obstruction complicated by parenchymal lung disorders, e.g., pneumonia or pulmonary edema, and/or extrapulmonary disorders, volume-time-regulated ventilators are preferable. Controlled ventilation is possible with appropriate sedation.

     Remember:

     Do not misinterpret blood gas levels during ventilation by failing to consider low baseline P_{aO_2} and high baseline P_{aCO_2} levels in these underlying disorders.
  3. The usual complications of mechanical ventilation may occur. Pressure trauma is common.

Prognosis

See Diagnosis.

Nursing Aspects

Weaning from mechanical ventilation is usually a long, trying process. Patients at this stage tend to develop hypersecretion and mucous plugging of airways, so that tracheotomy may be appropriate in some cases.

Definition

- Rapidly developing renal functional impairment, regardless of prior renal damage, that is potentially reversible following a repair phase
- Oliguria usually present; *total* anuria rare ($\frac{1}{4}$ to $\frac{1}{3}$ of all cases involve initial polyuria [urine output > 1000 mL/day] rather than oliguria.)
- Two forms should be distinguished, although they share the same etiologies, and may overlap considerably:
  - Functional, prerenal ARF
  - Parenchymal, intrarenal ARF (so-called tubular necrosis)

Etiology – Pathogenesis – Pathophysiology

- ARF is caused by renal ischemia due to imparment of blood supply to the kidney, and/or damage to the renal parenchyma by other factors (drugs, toxins, septicemia). Pathoanatomically, all degrees of tubular damage may be found, but the specific mechanisms responsible for the breakdown of filtration and continuation thereof have not yet been fully elucidated.
- ARF may be elicited by:
  - Cardiocirculatory shock
  - Dehydration, drug-induced hypovolemia, or hyponatremia
  - Septicemia
  - Peritonitis
  - Poisoning
  - Rhabdomyolysis
  - Disseminated intravascular clotting
  - Surgery or trauma

The most common precipitating factors were formerly shock and trauma, but septicemia has been implicated more and more frequently as the leading cause of ARF.

Diagnosis

- Clinical symptoms reflect the inability of the kidney to excrete *adequate* amounts of urine and nitrogenous waste products. The following capabilities are impaired:
  - Elimination of water
  - Elimination of electrolytes
  - Elimination of endogenous toxins and nitrogenous wastes
  - Elimination of exogenous toxins

The clinical and laboratory criteria of diagnosis when oliguria is the chief symptom are derived from these factors. Clinical symptoms do not develop until later.

Acute Renal Failure (ARF)

1. Laboratory:
   - Rapid increase of plasma creatinine levels
   - Decrease of creatinine clearance
   - Decrease of urine osmolality (U_{osm}) (early stage)
   - Urine/plasma osmotic ratio (U/P_{osm}) approaching 1:1
   - Decrease of free water clearance (H_2O) (early stage)
   - Hyperkalemia
   - Metabolic acidosis
2. Ultrasound: enlarged kidneys with rarefied cortex
3. Evidence of water overloading:
   - Pulmonary edema (early radiologic sign: "fluid lung")
   - Peripheral edema
   - Cerebral edema (clouded consciousness, enhanced neuromuscular irritability)

   Remember:

   In overt dehydration, it is not possible to differentiate functional ARF from ARF involving morphologic changes. Return of diuresis and renal function during and after rehydration clarifies the diagnosis.

- *Differential diagnosis:*
  - Distinction is to be made in the strictest sense between the following conditions and ARF: acute renal failure in the presence of chronic renal disease, acute glomerulonephritis with oliguria, and fulminant disease courses with renal involvement (particularly systemic immunologic disorders).
  - Bilateral renal vascular occlusion (usually with total anuria, which is rare in ARF; hematuria is common)
  - Postrenal kidney failure; localization:
    1. Suprapubic (bladder empty)
    2. Infrapubic (bladder full)

  Prior to initiation of treatment, these differential diagnostic possibilities must be ruled out by:
  - History
  - Complete clinical workup, including laboratory parameters
  - Ultrasound
  - Urinary bladder catheterization
  - Angiography (in appropriate cases)

Intensive Therapy

- Initial treatment is directed at eliminating known causes.
- Normalization of fluid balance is foremost. Prior to any further measures, provision must be made for:
  - Adequate circulating volume by administration of fluid and electrolytes
  - Adequate oncotic pressure of the plasma by administration of plasma/albumin

The dosages required vary, dependent on:
  - Clinical picture
  - Urine output
  - Central venous pressure
  - Serum albumin concentration

- After these possibilities have been exhausted:
  - Furosemide: start at 1–2 mg/kg and increase to 500–1000 mg as a short-term (30–60 min) IV infusion or ethacrynic acid 0.5–1 mg/kg b.w. If furosemide should fail, a trial of ethacrynic acid is justified.

Remember:
Premature administration of furosemide or ethacrynic acid may cause renal damage, especially in case of dehydration.
  - Dopamine 200–600 µg/min (has a beneficial effect on renal circulation)

Urine output initiated in this fashion can be maintained by furosemide 40–80 mg q 4–6 h or, alternatively, ethacrynic acid.

- If the above measures fail, hemodialysis is the procedure of choice, and should be initiated as early as possible (see below).

- Treatment of life-threatening hyperkalemia or hyperhydration before dialysis is available may be initiated by oral and rectal administration of potassium-binding synthetic resins (see p. 228) and/or IV infusions of glucose and insulin (see p. 229).

- Water may be eliminated by provoking diarrhea with sorbitol or mannitol (see p. 205).

- The following are signs of *overt* renal failure requiring immediate hemodialysis if initial therapeutic measures have failed, and the patient is acutely and severely ill:

  - Serum creatinine ≥ 3 mg/dL
  - Creatinine clearance < 25 mL/min
  - V_U < 20 mL/h, anuria
  - U_{osm} < 400 mosm/L
  - U/P_{osm} < 1.3

The technique of hemodialysis is described on p. 311.

Acute Renal Failure (ARF)

Complications

- The complications of ARF are:
  - Hyperkalemia
  - Water overloading with acute respiratory failure and heart failure
  - Gastrointestinal symptoms of uremia
  - Uremic coma due to ARF should not occur any more in view of the monitoring and therapeutic options now available.
- Complications of hemodialysis are described on p. 313.

Prognosis

- the short-term prognosis of ARF depends on the underlying disorder. Renal failure following sepsis, major surgery, or polytrauma, or in conjunction with multiple organic failure is lethal 80% of cases.
- Early recognition and treatment of dehydration and cardiocirculatory shock and preventive measures directed at these factors (input-output fluid balancing, protein replacement, hygienic precautions) are of prime importance.
  - Prompt initiation of hemodialysis once initial therapeutic possibilities have been exhausted assures a better prognosis.
- The long-term prognosis is favorable. Chronic disorders of renal function are of minor clinical relevance.

Disorders of Water and Sodium Homeostasis

Etiology – Pathogenesis

- Normal water and electrolyte homeostasis (euhydration) implies normal amounts and normal distribution of water and electrolytes throughout the entire organism and in individual fluid compartments. Disorders of the water and electrolyte system may involve deviations of content (imbalance) or abnormal distribution.

- Disorders of fluid balance:
  1. Hyperhydration refers to excessive accumulation of extracellular fluid due to an oversupply of sodium and water.
     - "Fluid overload" implies that water excess is the predominant or exclusive causative factor.
     - "Sodium overload" implies excessive sodium as the predominant causative factor.
  2. Dehydration refers to diminution of extracellular fluid due to reduction of sodium and water content.
     - "Simple dehydration" implies that diminished water content is exclusively or predominantly responsible.

- Disorders of distribution (dyshydration):
  Body fluids are abnormally distributed in the individual fluid compartments. The total water content may be normal, reduced, or elevated.

- Excessive sodium leads to hypertonic disorders, whereas too little sodium or an excess of water lead to hypotonic disorders.
  - Disorders of fluid balance and distribution are summarized in Table **5**.
  - Differentiation of disorders (EDH system) is summarized in Table **6**.

- Whether an isotonic or anisotonic deviation predominates usually depends more on the severity of the underlying disorder than on its etiology. For example, loss of extracellular fluid is followed initially by isotonic dehydration, until the deficiency becomes so excessive that osmotic regulation fails; then, the organism conserves relatively more water than sodium, leading to the most severe condition, hypotonic dehydration (depletion hyponatremia).

- Pathogenesis of disorders of water and electrolyte content involves only a few basic mechanisms (Fig. **4**):
  - Excessive output: If abnormal losses, e.g., due to vomiting, diarrhea, polyuria, or diaphoresis, are not compensated by a correspondingly increased intake, the predominance of output leads to deficiency.
  - Inadequate intake: Low intake for a long period cannot always be compensated by restricting excretion; the result is a deficit.
  - Excessive intake: If intake of water and electrolytes exceeds bodily requirements to such an extent that normally functioning

Disorders of Water and Sodium Homeostasis

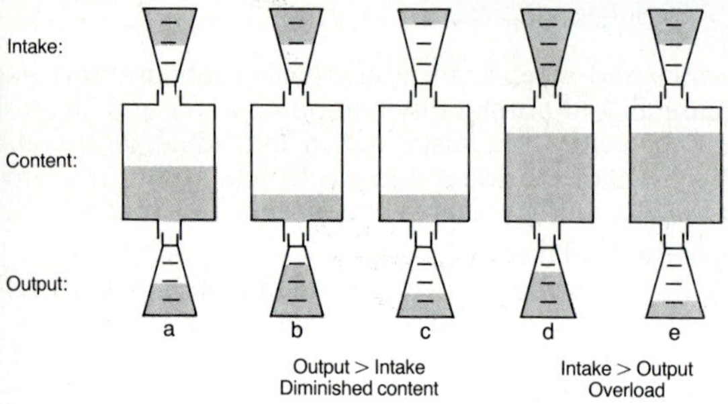

Fig. 4   Pathogenesis of disorders of fluid homeostasis

Table 5   Disorders of fluid balance (overview)

Disorders of water content	*Water depletion*			*Water excess*
		in isotonic solution		
Disorders of sodium content	*Sodium depletion*			*Sodium excess*
	=			=
	isotonic dehydratation			**isotonic hyperhydratation**
Tonicity disorders of extracellular fluid	water depletion (alone or predominantly)			predominantly excess of sodium
		Hyperosmolality (deficit of *free* water)		
	=			=
	hypertonic dehydratation			**hypertonic hyperhydratation**
	predominantly sodium depletion			excess of water (alone or predominantly)
		Hypoosmolality (excess of *free* water)		
	=			=
	hypotonic dehydratation			**hypotonic hyperhydratation**

Disorders of Water and Sodium Homeostasis

Table **6** Differentiation of disorders of water and sodium homeostasis by the EDH system (euhydration, dehydration, hyperhydration). N = normal, $\nearrow$ = elevated, $\searrow$ = diminished

EDH classification	Extracellular fluid: volume	osmolality	Sodium content	Diagnosis
Hypertonic dehydration	$\searrow$	$\nearrow$	N or $\searrow$	Simple water depletion (water deficit, normal Na content) / Predominantly water depletion (water deficit, diminished Na content)
Isotonic dehydration	$\searrow$	N	$\searrow$	Diminished extracellular volume (Na deficit in isotonic solution)
Hypotonic dehydration	$\searrow$	$\searrow$	$\searrow$	Predominantly Na depletion (water excess, Na deficit)
Euhydration	N	N	N	
Hypotonic hyperhydration	$\nearrow$	$\searrow$	N or $\nearrow$	Simple excess of water, normal Na supply / Predominantly excess of water (water excess, enhanced Na supply)
Isotonic hyperhydration	$\nearrow$	N	$\nearrow$	Enhanced extracellular volume (excess Na in isotonic solution)
Hypertonic hyperhydration	$\nearrow$	$\nearrow$	$\nearrow$	Predominantly oversupply of Na (water depletion, enhanced availability of Na)

Disorders of Water and Sodium Homeostasis

excretory mechanisms are overtaxed, disorders may occur. An example is improperly balanced IV infusion therapy.

– Impaired excretory output: Disorders of normal processes of elimination of water and electrolytes may lead to excesses thereof even if the intake is "normal." Typical examples include renal failure with oligoanuria, congestive heart failure, hepatic failure, and conditions involving inadequate secretion of ADH (antidiuretic hormone).

• Specific causes of disorders of sodium-water homeostasis are listed under Differential Diagnosis.

Table 7   Criteria for identification of disorders of fluid and electrolyte homeostasis (findings)

	Dehydration	Hyperhydration
History	GI losses, polyuria, fever, thirst	renal failure with oliguria, prior infusions
Clinical findings		
Dampness of skin and mucous membranes	dryness	unremarkable
Tissue turgor	diminished	enhanced
Edema		evident
Change of body weight	rapid loss	rapid gain
Urinary output per unit time	diminished*	unremarkable
Central venous pressure	diminished	elevated
Arterial circulation	tachycardia, vasoconstriction, hypotension	elevation of blood pressure
Pulmonary findings	unremarkable	fluid lung, alveolar edema
Laboratory findings		
Total plasma protein	↗	↘
Hemoglobin	↗	↘
Hematocrit		
Serum osmolality		hypertonic, isotonic, hypotonic
Serum sodium		

* Assuming normal renal function and no osmotic diuresis. Oligo-anuric renal failure involves oliguria with hyperhydration, and osmotic diuresis involves polyuria with dehydration.

Diagnosis

- Monitoring of fluid homeostasis is based on clinical findings, serial assessments of body weight and CVP at regular intervals, and certain laboratory tests. In routine practice, clinical evidence, including checks of body weight and CVP, are most important in evaluation of fluid homeostasis with respect to euhydration, hyperhydration, dehydration, and dyshydration.

- Clinical and laboratory chemical parameters for evaluation of fluid homeostasis are summarized in Tables **7** and **8**.

Table **8**   Criteria for evaluation of water and electrolyte homeostasis (overview)

Clinical symptoms:

Tissue turgidity
Moisture of skin and mucous membranes
Edema
Pulmonary findings
Signs of vasoconstriction
Behavior of blood pressure

Clinical and laboratory findings:

Changes in body weight
Urinary output per unit time and urinary osmolarity
Serum protein concentration, hemoglobin, hematocrit
Sodium and potassium concentrations in serum and urine
Serum osmolarity
Central venous pressure

Signs of hypovolemia:

Diminished tissue turgor, dry skin and mucous membranes, signs of cutaneous vasoconstriction
Rapid weight loss
Low urinary output with high osmolarity
Increase of serum protein concentration and hemoglobin or hematocrit
Central venous pressure low from the start, or decreasing during the course

Signs of hypervolemia:

Enhanced tissue turgor, edema, tachypnea, arterial hypoxemia; pulmonary rales and radiographic evidence of fluid lung are optional
Rapid weight gain
Decrease of serum protein concentration and hemoglobin or hematocrit
Central venous pressure high from the start, or increasing during the course

Disorders of Water and Sodium Homeostasis

Differential Diagnosis

- Disorders of fluid homeostasis are classified according to the EDH system (euhydration, dehydration, hyperhydration).
  Dehydration and hyperhydration may be further subdivided into isotonic, hypotonic, and hypertonic forms, depending on the osmolality of the extracellular fluid. Since the osmotic pressure of the extracellular fluid depends chiefly upon the sodium level, the relative increase or decrease of water and sodium is a sufficiently accurate parameter for assessment of osmotic behavior in clinical evaluation.

  A disorder is referred to as isotonic if deficit or excess of water and sodium are proportionate. In hypertonic disorders, a water deficit or excess of sodium predominates. Hypotonic disorders result from a sodium deficit or excess of water.

- Causes of disorders of fluid-sodium homeostasis:
  1. Deficit of water and sodium due to:
     - impaired intake of water in:
       - a) unconsciousness
       - b) weakness, physical disability
       - c) impaired swallowing
       - d) inflammations or caustic damage to the GI tract
       - e) psychosis
     - febrile states, prolonged transsudation
     - protracted vomiting
     - diarrhea
     - villous adenoma of the colon
     - gastrointestinal drainage
     - intestinal fistulas or stomas
     - drainage of body cavities
     - diuretics
     - osmotic diuresis due to hyperglycemia
     - postobstructive polyuria
     - chronic renal failure with polyuria
     - polyuric phase of acute renal failure
     - chronic nephritis with salt-losing nephropathy
     - adrenal cortical failure
     - diabetes insipidus

2. Excess of water and sodium due to:
   - Acute oligoanuric renal failure
   - Chronic oliguric renal failure
   - Decompensated congestive heart failure
   - Decompensated hepatic failure
   - Excessive administration of water or sodium (e.g., overinfusion)
   - Hypothyroidism
   - Excessive secretion of ADH, as in:
     a) Malignancies (bronchogenic carcinoma, etc.)
     b) CNS disorders
     c) Chronic pulmonary diseases

Initial Care

- Obvious dehydration with clinical evidence of exsiccosis: infusion of isotonic electrolytes (physiologic saline or balanced electrolytes in Ringer's lactate), starting with about 1000 mL/h. Initial rehydration by infusion of saline is also the best first step in treatment of diabetic coma.
- Clear evidence of hyperhydration with complications (see above): injection of a fast-acting diuretic, e.g., furosemide 40 mg IV

Continuing Care

- Treatment of disorders of fluid balance in ICU patients is part of balanced fluid administration.
- Treatment of dyshydration is directed at the cause:
  - Replacement of albumin and treatment of the cause in hypoproteinemia
  - Drainage of effusions in body cavities
  - Treatment of congestive heart failure
  - Treatment of intestinal obstruction
  - Treatment of peritonitis
  - Treatment of pancreatitis
  - Treatment of acute respiratory failure
  - Treatment of septicemia

Disorders of Water and Sodium Homeostasis

Complications

- Complications of dehydration:
  - Circulatory collapse with tachycardia, hypotension; in severe cases, hypovolemic shock
  - Functional renal failure
  - Fever
  - Restlessness, confusion, clouded consciousness; in severe cases, coma with irreversible organic brain damage
- Complications of hyperhydration:
  - Hypervolemia with acute heart failure in severe cases, intraalveolar pulmonary edema
  - Acute respiratory failure due to interstitial pulmonary edema (fluid lung)
  - Brain edema with seizures, clouded consciousness, or unconsciousness
- Dyshydration due to sequestration of fluid may be difficult to detect. Suspicion of diversion of fluid to a third space is based on typical clinical findings with evidence of volume depletion, and particularly of diminished circulating blood volume (hypovolemia), despite balanced or even positive input-output data on fluid balance.

Disorders of Potassium Homeostasis

Etiology – Pathogenesis – Pathophysiology

- Disorders of potassium homeostasis are due to diminution of the potassium content (potassium deficit), enhancement of the potassium content (potassium excess), or disorders of potassium distribution between the intracellular and extracellular spaces. In practice, the most important single factor in etiology of disorders of potassium distribution is alteration of blood pH: Alkalosis causes potassium to enter the cells, whereas acidosis causes it to leave them.
- Causes of disorders of potassium content:
  1. Potassium deficit:
     - Enteric loss (vomiting, diarrhea, gastrointestinal drainage or fistulas)
     - Sequestration of potassium in third spaces (intestinal obstruction, peritonitis, pancreatitis)
     - Renal loss (saluretic drugs, polyuria due to nephropathy or osmotic diuresis)
     - Deficient administration in artificial alimentation
     - Abuse of laxatives
  2. Potassium excess:
     - Impaired elimination (acute or chronic renal failure, potassium-sparing diuretics in renal failure)
     - Overinfusion
     - Massive tissue trauma in the presence of renal failure
     - Adrenal cortical insufficiency
- Causes of disorders of potassium distribution:
  - Hyperkalemia in metabolic acidosis
  - Hypokalemia in metabolic alkalosis
  - Hyperkalemia due to massive intravascular hemolysis
  - Hyperkalemia in initial stages of acute digitalis poisoning with large overdoses

Diagnosis

- Clinical findings:
  - Clinical symptoms of potassium deficiency reflect disorders of neuromuscular excitability: adynamia, attenuated reflexes and muscle tone, paresthesias, gastrointestinal atony, voiding difficulties, impairment of formation and conduction of cardiac excitation (arrhythmias, S-T depression, flattened T waves, prolonged Q-T interval, T-U fusion.
  - Clinical symptoms of excessive potassium are derived from formation and conduction of cardiac excitation waves (arrhythmia, high T waves, widened QRS complexes).
  - Clinical signs of disorders of potassium content are nonspecific; in ICU patients they tend to be masked by other symptoms.

Disorders of Potassium Homeostasis

- ECG alterations (Fig. **5**) may provide clues to disorders of potassium homeostasis, but electrocardiography is inadequate for monitoring this parameter due to lack of specificity and sensitivity.

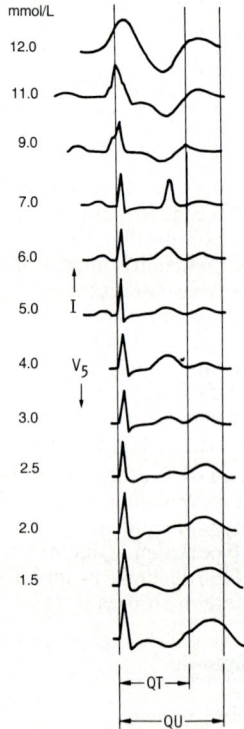

Hyperkalemic arrhythmias	mmol/L
Sinus bradycardia	12.0
1st degree AV block	11.0
AV-nodal rhythm	
Idioventricular rhythm	9.0
Ventricular tachycardia	
Ventricular fibrillation	7.0
Ventricular arrest	
	6.0
	5.0
Normal ECG	
	4.0
	3.0
Hypokalemic arrhythmias	2.5
Ventricular extrasystoles	
Atrial tachycardia	2.0
AV-nodal tachycardia	
Ventricular tachycardia	1.5
Ventricular fibrillation	

Fig. **5**   ECG alterations in disorders of potassium homeostasis

- Serum potassium levels:
  - Standard parameter for assessment of potassium balance is the serum potassium concentration.
  - The relationship of serum potassium levels to current potassium content depends on the potassium capacity. The potassium capacity is defined as the sum of all intracellular anions or other chemical groups capable of binding potassium. The potassium capacity is a function of the total cellular mass (including the erythrocytes) and the glycogen content. Disorders of potassium homeostasis may result from changes of potassium capacity despite normal potassium content (tissue breakdown, hemolysis, malnutrition, glycogen formation), or from alterations of potassium content despite unchanged potassium capacity. If the potassium content is less than the potassium capacity, there is a potassium deficit. Potassium content in excess of the capacity is equivalent to potassium overload.

    The concentration of potassium in serum is a specific parameter for the relationship of potassium content to capacity, provided that potassium is distributed normally between the extracellular and intracellular compartments. Potassium content in excess of capacity = hyperkalemia; potassium content below the capacity = hypokalemia.

    In the plot of potassium content (abscissa) versus serum potassium (ordinate), the slope becomes steeper above 3 mmol/L potassium in serum, indicating greater sensitivity of the potassium level to changes in content in the hyperkalemic range. Potassium content exceeding the capacity by +5% increases the serum potassium level by 1 mmol/L. In the hypokalemic range the curve flattens, and changes in potassium content have less and less effect on measured serum levels. The content must decrease by 10–15% to cause the potassium levels to drop by 1 mmol/L.
  - Serum potassium levels lose their specifity as indicators of the potassium content if the distribution of potassium between the intracellular and extracellular spaces is disrupted. The best-known example of a disorder of distribution is the interdependence of the ratio of intra- to extracellular potassium and pH. Change of the concentration of H^+ ions results in counterchange of the gradient of intra- to extracellular potassium.
  - Estimation of potassium content on the basis of the serum potassium level as a function of arterial pH (Table 9).
  - Rule-of-thumb: A shift in pH by 0.1 points causes serum potassium levels to change by about 0.6 mmol/L on the average; variations are considerable (0.4 to 1.2 mmol/L), the extent of change of potassium concentration being a direct function of the concentration.
  - Some reference values are listed in Table 10.

Disorders of Potassium Homeostasis

Table 9   Inferences concerning potassium content based on serum potassium levels

Serum potassium concentration	Potassium content
Normokalemia, normal pH	Normal, possibly slightly enhanced or diminished
Hypokalemia, normal pH	Potassium deficiency
Hyperkalemia, normal pH	Potassium excess
Normokalemia, alkalosis	Potassium excess
Hyperkalemia, alkalosis	Marked potassium excess
Hypokalemia, alkalosis	Equivocal
Normokalemia, acidosis	Potassium deficiency
Hypokalemia, acidosis	Severe potassium deficiency
Hyperkalemia, acidosis	Equivocal

Table 10   Influence of pH on serum potassium concentration

pH	7.0	7.2	7.4	7.6
Potassium	4.7 mmol/L $\longrightarrow$	3.7 mmol/L $\longrightarrow$	3.0 mmol/L $\longleftarrow$	2.3 mmol/L
	6.2 mmol/L $\longrightarrow$	4.9 mmol/L $\longrightarrow$	4.0 mmol/L $\longleftarrow$	3.2 mmol/L
	8.0 mmol/L $\longrightarrow$	6.2 mmol/L $\longrightarrow$	5.0 mmol/L $\longleftarrow$	3.8 mmol/L
	10.0 mmol/L $\longrightarrow$	7.3 mmol/L $\longrightarrow$	6.0 mmol/L $\longleftarrow$	4.5 mmol/L

- Potassium in urine: Urinary potassium concentrations below 10 mmol/L and decrease of potassium clearance to less than 5 ml/min are suggestive of a potassium deficit.

Immediate Care

- Adequate treatment of disorders of potassium balance is usually feasible only under in-hospital conditions. Exceptions:
  - Hypokalemic cardiocirculatory arrest: Slow IV injection of 15 mmol KCl over a 5 min period
  - Severe ECG changes or cardiocirculatory complications in case of known hyperkalemia: IV infusion of a glucose-insulin mixture (500 mL 10% glucose + 20–30 U of standard insulin) within 30 min.

Continuing Care

- Restoration of potassium homeostasis (see p. 228).
- In hyperkalemia, extraction of potassium by extracorporeal hemodialysis or cationic ion exchange resins
  - Cationic ion exchange resins may be administered orally or rectally; they bind potassium in exchange for sodium or calcium. The effect is enhanced by simultaneous administration of sorbitol to elicit osmotic diarrhea.
- In hypokalemia, potassium replacement by infusion (see Potassium Balancing, p. 228).

Complications

- Life-threatening complications: cardiac arrhythmias; in extreme cases, ventricular fibrillation or asystole
- ECG changes are inadequate for overall monitoring of potassium balance, but may provide clues of immediate danger in severe hypo- or hyperkalemia.
  Remember:
  Malignant cardiac arrhythmias may develop abruptly even without prior electrocardiographic signs.
- The danger posed by hyperkalemia depends on the etiology. Experience has shown hyperkalemia due to intravascular hemolysis to be tolerated better than hyperkalemia due to other causes.

Phosphate Depletion Syndrome

Definition

- Phosphate depletion refers to massive reduction of phosphate content due to functional disorders or organic complications. Hypophosphatemia does not necessarily imply phosphate depletion, since there is no linear relationship between serum phosphate and total phosphate [except in RBCs (red blood cells)]. Genuine phosphate depletion is a rare, but critical, condition.

Etiology – Pathogenesis

- A massive phosphate deficit may result from a negative input-output balance or from abnormal phosphate distribution. Pathogenetic mechanisms that may give rise to hypophosphatemia, and thus be potential causes of a phosphate depletion syndrome, are:
  - Phosphate binding within the GI tract by large amounts of antacids
  - Severe burns (wasting)
  - Diabetic ketoacidosis or metabolic acidosis (disorders of distribution)
  - Alcohol abuse
  - Hyperalimentation, nutritional recovery syndrome (acute anabolic state)
  - Parenteral alimentation for more than 10 days, particularly if fructose is the predominant component (wasting and disorders of distribution)

Diagnosis

- Hypophosphatemia is the leading symptom. Phosphate levels below 1 mg/dL, markedly altered amounts in urine, and abnormal phosphate clearance are suggestive of a clinically significant disorder. Other routine laboratory parameters are irrelevant.
- Clinically significant disorders lead to organ dysfunction:
  - Diminished synthesis of 2,3-DPG (diphosphoglyceric acid) and ATP (adenosene triphosphate) by RBCs and leftward shift of the O_2 binding curve
  - Impaired WBC function
  - Impaired platelet function
  - Neurologic deficiencies
  - Rhabdomyolysis
  - Impairment of hepatocellular function
  - Impairment of renal function
  - Congestive heart failure

- Neurologic deficiencies are the most obvious clinical signs:
  - Clouding of consciousness, loss of consciousness
  - Apathy, weakness
  - Palsies
  - Delayed awakening following long-term sedation, other causes being ruled out

Diagnosis is still based largely on exclusion, but even suspicion of phosphate depletion in conjunction with laboratory data requires appropriate therapy. The diagnosis is often made retrospectively following response to treatment.

Remember:

Phosphate depletion may be prevented by advance replacement.

Intensive Therapy

- Phosphate replacement with:
  - Potassium phosphate buffer
  - Sodium phosphate buffer

For details and subsequent procedures, see p. 230.

Prognosis

- Favorable, provided replacement is adequate and initiated early
- Tendency of neurologic symptoms to resolve rapidly

Disorders of Acid-Base Metabolism

Etiology – Pathogenesis – Pathophysiology

- Abnormalities of acid-base balance result from a deficit or excess of acidic or basic valences that cannot be compensated by the body's buffer systems or renal or pulmonary excretory mechanisms. The problem is a quantitative one for the rapidly functioning buffer systems and pulmonary regulation, but for renal mechanisms, which act over a period of hours, time too becomes important.

- Primary respiratory disorders develop when release of CO_2 by the lungs occurs at a slower or faster rate than its production (respiratory acidosis or respiratory alkalosis, respectively).

- Metabolic disorders result from an oversupply of acids or bases by endogenous production, exogenous supply, pathologic losses, or inadequate renal elimination.

- Typical causes of acid-base disorders in ICU patients are:
  1. Causes of metabolic acidosis:
     - Shock
     - "Low cardiac output" syndromes
     - Cardiocirculatory arrest
     - Diabetic acidosis (ketoacidosis, lactacidosis)
     - Chronic and/or acute renal failure
     - End-stage hepatic failure
     - Loss of alkaline intestinal juices (severe diarrhea, intestinal drains or fistulas, GI stomas)
     - Poisoning
  2. Causes of metabolic alkalosis:
     - Loss of acidic gastric juices (severe vomiting, gastric drainage via tube)
     - Overcorrection of acidosis
     - Rapid diminution of pCO_2 in case of metabolically compensated respiratory acidosis (posthypercapnic alkalosis)
     - Severely decompensated end-stage hepatic failure
     - Diuretics (furosemide, ethacrynic acid)
     - Potassium deficiency with hypokalemia and extracellular acidosis due to unequal distribution
  3. Causes of respiratory acidosis:
     - Bronchopulmonary disease with obstructive or restrictive impairment of ventilation
     - Central depression of respiration with hypoventilation
     - Peripheral respiratory paralysis
     - Airways obstruction
  4. Causes of respiratory alkalosis:
     - Mechanical hyperventilation
     - Fever
     - Cerebrocranial trauma and other brain disorders

Disorders of Acid-Base Metabolism

Diagnosis

- The clinical signs of alkalosis and acidosis are nonspecific; in ICU patients they are usually masked by other symptoms. Exceptions are deep Kussmaul respirations in spontaneously breathing patients with metabolic acidosis and the hyperventilation syndrome as causes of respiratory alkalosis.

- Diagnosis is based on analysis of arterial blood or capillary blood from the hyperemic ear lobe for pH, pCO_2, and HCO_3 concentration. Differentiation of primary respiratory from metabolic disorders is complicated by the fact that the actual bicarbonate concentration as expressed by the Henderson-Hasselbalch equation is modified by primary changes of pCO_2. To take this into account, the notion of standard bicarbonate (i.e., plasma bicarbonate at $pCO_2 = 40$ mmHg and $37°C$) has been devised. Base deviations and base excess denote the deviation of a measured buffer base concentration from normal values at $pCO_2 = 40$ mmHg and pH = 7.40.

Differential Diagnosis

- The most widely used scheme for differention of disorders of acid-base balance is shown in Table **11**.
Remember:
This diagram is too crude to describe complex disorders adequately. Complex disorders are frequently misinterpreted as partially or completely compensated simple ones. Still, the scheme

Table **11**   Differentiation of disorders of acid-base equilibrium

Diagnosis	pH	pCO_2	Standard bicarbonate	Base excess
Metabolic acidosis				
– decompensated	↘	↔	↘	negative
– compensated	↘↓	↔↓	↘	negative
Metabolic alkalosis				
– decompensated	↗	↔	↗	positive
– compensated	↗↑	↗↑	↗	positive
Respiratory acidosis				
– decompensated	↘	↗	↔	↔
– compensated	↘↑	↗	↗↑	positive
Respiratory alkalosis				
– decompensated	↗	↘		↔
– kompensated	↗↑	↘↘	↘↓	negative

Disorders of Acid-Base Metabolism

serves as a convenient guideline for making therapeutic decisions, since as a rule only obviously decompensated deviations ($pH_a < 7.30$, $pH_a > 7.50$) require active treatment. Compensated or mildly decompensated disorders will respond to autoregulatory processes once the underlying condition has been adequately treated.

Immediate Care

- Immediate therapy without analysis of acid-base status is indicated only in cardiocirculatory arrest: administration of sodium bicarbonate (see p. 224).

Continuing Therapy

- Daily computation of the acid-base input-output balance.

Complications

- Respiratory alkalosis during mechanical ventilation may result in arterial hypotension, neurologic symptoms, seizures, and coma.
- Metabolic acidosis may elicit ventricular fibrillation.
- Metabolic acidosis has a depressant effect on the cardiocirculatory system (diminution of cardiac output, inadequate response to catecholamines, hypotension, cardiac rhythm disorders).
  Remember:
  This holds true only for extreme acidosis, in animal experiments starting at pH values below 7.0. The critical pH_a levels in ICU patients are assumed to be < 7.3 in cardiovascular disorders and < 7.2 in ketoacidosis.
- Respiratory acidosis can lead to clouding of consciousness and coma (acute exacerbation or hypoventilation-hypercapnia syndrome during O_2 administration to patients with obstructive airways disease and chronic respiratory failure).

Definition

- Hypothermia denotes lowering of the rectal body temperature to below 35°C, moderate hypothermia to about 32°C, and severe hypothermia to below 32°C.

Etiology – Pathogenesis – Pathophysiology

- *Pathogenesis:*
  - Protracted exposure to cold; disorders of thermoregulation
  - Elderly individuals more susceptible (age-dependent impairment of thermoregulation)
  - Children more susceptible (poor insulation by skin and subcutaneous fat)
  - Hypothyroidism, predisposing to hypothermia (impaired heat production)
- *Etiology:*
  - Unconsciousness due to exogenous poisoning with hypnotic or psychotropic drugs (e.g., barbiturates, phenothiazines, benzodiazepines, tricyclic antidepressants) or ethanol
  - Ketoacidotic coma
  - Prolonged immersion in cold water, e.g., after accidents (maximum survival time in 15°C water 12 h, in 10°C water 5 h, in 0–5°C water 30–90 min)
  - Severe brain damage with loss of thermoregulation capability; hypothermia is a symptom of dissociated brain death
- *Pathophysiology:* The following disorders develop as the degree of hypothermia increases:
  - Impairment of consciousness and loss of reflexes; unconsciousness in severe hypothermia
  - Cardiac conduction disorders (ECG: typical J wave), bradycardia, cardiac arrhythmias; in extreme cases, ventricular fibrillation
  - Hypotension
  - Infrequent, weak respiration
  - Cutaneous swelling due to subcutaneous edema
    Metabolic complications with acidosis, hyperglycemia, enhancement of serum CPK activity

Diagnosis

- Measurement of rectal temperature with special thermometer (special model for premature infants or electrothermometer)

Hypothermia

Immediate Care

- In cardiocirculatory arrest: cardiopulmonary resuscitation
  Remember:
  Resuscitation may be successful even at body temperatures below 25°C or following prolonged anoxia (slowed metabolism, diminished oxygen requirements, better tolerance of anoxia).

Therapy

- Administration of warmth (see p. 326).

Complications

- See Pathophysiology
- Coma
- Cardiocirculatory shock
- Ventricular fibrillation at body temperatures below 28–30°C
- Metabolic decompensation

Definition

- Progressive to complete loss of CNS function due to intra- or extracerebral disorders. A comatose patient cannot be wakened; coma staging is based on clinical and neurologic evidence.
- Coma staging:
  1. Patient cannot be wakened.
     Specific avoidance responses to painful stimuli, reflexes, and autonomic functions largely intact
  2. Nonspecific or absent avoidance responses to painful stimuli; impairment of autonomic function
     Brainstem reflexes depend on site of damage:
     - Diencephalic lesions: pupils moderately dilated, reaction to light intact; respiration depressed
     - Mesencephalic syndrome: pupils dilated, reactions to light greatly diminished, bulbi divergent, oculocephalic reflexes absent, but corneal reflexes intact; pyramidal tract signs positive, respiration often machine-like
  3. Complete absence of defensive and motoric responses and brainstem reflexes; severe impairment of autonomic functions and respiration
  4. No reaction whatever; no reflex responses; no spontaneous respiration; autonomic processes severely impaired
     Remember:
     Precise description and/or staging of the state of consciousness and coma is essential for evaluation of the course and for therapeutic decisions. It helps avoid misunderstandings, especially on an interdisciplinary level.
- Acute exogenous poisoning may give rise to combinations of neurologic symptoms that elude the staging classification and that do not match well, e.g., extension spasms and low-grade coma. Such combinations may provide *one* initial differential diagnostic clue as to the cause of the coma.

Etiology – Pathogenesis

- Primary cerebral coma
  Primary cerebral coma results from structural damage to brain tissue, and the neurologic defects depend on the site of the lesion and anatomic factors. Most common causes: head injuries, cerebrovascular accidents
- Postischemic-anoxic coma due to brain damage *from* cardiopulmonary resuscitation or extreme hypoxia
- Hypoxic coma, i.e., loss of consciousness *during* manifest hypoxia

Coma of Indeterminate Origin

- Primary toxic coma:
  - Acute exogenous poisoning
  - Metabolic comas
  - Endocrine comas

  In metabolic-toxic coma, development of neurologic defects depends on the sensitivity of the affected parts of the brain.

  Remember:

  Acute exogenous poisoning is the most frequent nontraumatic cause of comas; comas of cerebrovascular origin rank next.

Differential Diagnosis

- Before physical examination, vital functions must be secured in accordance with the ABC rule:
  - A: Open the *A*irway.
  - B: Maintain *B*reathing.
  - C: Maintain *C*irculation.
- Elicit the case history. Assistants should be charged with interviewing companions, transportation personnel, physicians, relatives, and friends capable of providing information.
- The basic examination protocol, parts of which may be carried out concurrently, permits preliminary diagnostic assessment:
  - Dipstick tests: Hyper- vs. hypoglycemia
  - Cutaneous findings:

    Blisters in sleeping-pill overdosage

    Dry, warm skin in acute hyperthyroidism

    Cutaneous hepatic stigmas

    Uremic skin discoloration
  - Fetid breath:

    Alcohol

    Uremia

    Hepatic disease

    Acetonemia

    Garlic-like in poisoning with organic phosphates

    Other odors typical of certain poisonings
  - Respiration:

    Infrequent: poisoning with central sedatives or opiates; myxedema

    Frequent: hyperthyroidism, mesencephalic lesions

    Kussmaul respiration: Ketoacidosis, uremic acidosis

    Cheyne-Stokes respiration: elevated intracranial pressure

    Machine-like respiration: mesencephalic lesions

– The basic neurologic workup should always proceed according to the same protocol, and should include:

a) *Skeletal muscles:*

Hemiplegia with corresponding asymmetry of muscular stretching reflexes and unilaterally positive Babinski reflex: focal cerebral lesions

Remember:

Small intracerebral hemorrhages and ischemia located near the midline do not necessarily give rise to hemiplegic symptoms.

– Involuntary hyperkinesia: more likely in metabolic or toxic lesions
– Muscular fibrillation: organic phosphate poisoning
– Enhanced muscle tone in hypertension: brain stem lesions
– Muscle tone and motility as in deep sleep: barbiturate or tranquilizer poisoning
– stereotyped rolling, wiping, and beating movements: primary subcortical cerebral lesions

b) *Pupillary muscles:*

– Miosis: parasympathomimetic or sympatholytic drugs, morphine, pontine hemorrhage, organic phosphate poisoning
– Mydriasis: parasympatholytic agents (e.g., atropine), hypnotic drugs
– Intermediate size with negative response to light: mesencephalic lesions
– Unilateral dilation: temporal lobe herniation

c) *Extrinsic ocular motility:*

– Impairment of reflexes is more strongly indicative of a structural lesion than of a metabolic disorder.

• Secondary examinations:

– Laboratory tests:

Blood sugar
Electrolytes
Blood gases and acid-base status
Serum transaminases
NH_3
Nitrogenous wastes in blood
Hematology
Thyroid hormones
Toxicology screening tests (see p. 192)
Blood alcohol level
Ketone bodies
Creatinine phosphokinase (markedly elevated in barbiturate poisoning)

– Plain abdominal films (bromic carbamide is opaque on x-ray)

Coma of Indeterminate Origin

- If the origin of the coma is not revealed by the above testing, further elucidation by specific tests is required, preferably in collaboration with a neurologist.
  - Fundoscopy
  - Specific neurologic testing, e.g., of oculovestibular reflexes
  - CAT scan
  - EEG with attention to the following questions: Signs of lateralization
    Overall pathology
    Specific pathology, especially "burst suppression" patterns
  - Spinal tap if meningoencephalitis or subarachnoid hemorrhage are suspected

Remember:
Generalized seizures frequently accompany poisoning by:
  - Diphenhydramine
  - Methaqualone
  - Carbromal
  - INH (isonicotinic acid hydrazide)
  - Anticholinergic drugs
  - Quinidine
  - Strychnine

Treatment

- Intensive monitoring and intensive care
- Specific treatment of the basic condition or most likely cause of the coma.
  - Gastric lavage or forced diuresis are contraindicated until the diagnosis has been confirmed

Remember:
Trial gastric lavage and forced diuresis may be fatal in primary cerebral coma.

Complications

- Hypoxic brain damage if basic procedures to assure vital functions are neglected
- Brain herniation following premature lumbar puncture done without or for wrong indication

Etiology – Pathogenesis

- Insulin deficiency in controlled diabetes mellitus due to:
  - Intercurrent infection
  - Acute gastroenteritis
  - Operation and/or accidents
  - Severe dietary mistakes
  - Psychological strain
- Coma as initial manifestation of previously undiagnosed diabetes mellitus

Clinical Findings – Diagnosis

- The coma results from hyperosmolality and ketonemia due to hyperglycemia, the chain of events being osmotic diuresis, dehydration, metabolic acidosis, and ionic shifts.
- Clinical findings:
  - Marked dehydration
  - Facial flushing
  - Hypotension
  - Tachycardia
  - Kussmaul respiration
  - Acetone odor
  - Hyporeflexia or areflexia
  - Diabetic pseudoperitonitis (in some cases)
- Laboratory findings:
  - Hyperglycemia (400–1000 mg/dL)
  - Metabolic acidosis
  - Evidence of ketone bodies
  - Plasma osmolality increase (to above 310 mOsm/L)

Differential Diagnosis

- Hyperglycemia without ketoacidosis occurs in:
  - Diabetic hyperosmolar coma (see p. 157)
  - Myocardial infarction
  - Pancreatitis
  - Cerebrovascular accidents
  - Post-stress metabolism following surgery and trauma.
- Hypoglycemic coma

Therapy

- See p. 241.

Prognosis

- Early onset of treatment is critical, especially with regard to restoring fluid and electrolyte equilibrium. Total lethality still exceeds 20%.

Hyperosmolar Nonketotic Coma

Etiology – Pathogenesis

- As in diabetic coma, but without ketoacidosis
- Iatrogenic by IV infusion (e.g., of highly concentrated dextrose solutions or inadequate amounts of water)
- Central disorders of osmoregulation

Clinical Signs – Diagnosis

- Signs of dehydration with hypovolemia dominate the clinical picture:
  - High-grade exsiccosis
  - Generalized seizures
  - Tachycardia
  - Hypotension
- Laboratory diagnosis:
  - Hyperglycemia (600–1200 mg/dL)
  - Serum potassium diminished, serum sodium normal, slightly elevated, or diminished
  - Markedly increased plasma osmolality (in excess of 360 mOsm/L)
  - No evidence of ketone bodies
  - Metabolic acidosis absent or very mild

Differential Diagnosis

- As in ketotic diabetic coma
- Central nervous seizures due to other causes

Therapy

- See p. 241.

Etiology – Pathogenesis

- Dietary mistakes or insulin overdosage
- Functional hyperinsulinism
- Islet-cell adenoma or extrapancreatic insulin-producing tumor
- Endocrine disorders
- Severe hepatic parenchymal disease
- Acute exogenous poisoning by alcohol, carbon tetrachloride, strychnine, or *Amanita phalloides* mushrooms
- Iatrogenic by IV infusion therapy (e.g., abrupt changes of dextrose or insulin dosage or IV administration of solutions containing dextrose and insulin)

Clinical Signs – Diagnosis

- Clinical signs:
  - Pallor, diaphoresis
  - Tachycardia
  - Hypotension
  - Enhanced excitation of reflexes
  - Cerebral seizures
- Laboratory evidence:
  - Hypoglycemia

Therapy

- See p. 241.
  Remember:
  In case of difficulty in deciding whether hypo- or hyperglycemic coma is involved, inject 40–80 mL 20% D/W IV. In hypoglycemia, this usually brings about rapid improvement.

Definition

- Acute onset of life-threatening exacerbation of symptoms of hyper-thyroidism

Etiology – Pathogenesis

- Untreated or inadequately treated hyperthyroidism
- Postoperative state
- Stressful situations of any type
- Toxic thyroid adenoma
- Radioiodide treatment and radiographic contrast dyes containing iodine
Remember:
Verification of venous catheter position by means of contrast dyes containing iodine are contraindicated in patients with known history of hyperthyroidism.

Diagnosis

- Clinical symptoms:
  - Tachycardia, tachyarrhythmia, pulse rate > 150/min
  - Motor and psychological agitation to the point of delirium
  - Hyperpyrexia
  - Dehydration
  - Initially, increasing blood pressure, with wide amplitude and all signs of circulatory hyperkinesia; later, hypotension to the point of shock
  - Oliguria
  - Vomiting, diarrhea
- Laboratory evidence:
  - Serum T_3 and T_4 levels markedly elevated
  - Cholesterol diminished
  - Alkaline phosphatase increased
  - BUN elevated
  - Hyponatremia
- *Differential Diagnosis:*
  - Neuropsychiatric disorders (particularly at onset)
  - Toxic comas of other origin

Definitive Therapy

- Intensive monitoring and intensive care
- Sedation with phenobarbital, promethazine-HCl, or diazepam
- Beta-adrenergic inhibitors, preferably continuously via IV infusion pump
- Hydrocortisone 50–100 mg/8 h IV
- Propylthiouracil: controlling dose 200–600 mg daily in divided doses; maintenance 50–200 mg daily
- High-calorie alimentation
- Hyperthermic blankets
- O_2 administration
- Plasmapheresis may be appropriate in life-threatening cases that fail to respond to conservative treatment. However, it appears to be effective only if 4–6 L can be exchanged.

Complications

- Heart failure
- Acute renal failure with oligoanuria
- Marked hepatic parenchymal damage, in severe cases with hepatic atrophy coma
- Cranial nerve palsies
- Myopathies
- Acute respiratory failure

Prognosis

- If appropriate therapy is initiated early, the lethality is less than 20%.

Follow-up Treatment

- Tapering of cortisone and propylthiouracil
- Readjustment of antithyroid medication

Definition

- Coma due to failure of thyroid function, with (or, rarely, without) myxedema

Etiology – Pathogenesis

- End stage of primary hypothyroidism
- Sequela of thyroiditis
- Sequela of antithyroid treatment

Diagnosis

- Clinical signs:
  - Often goiter and macroglossia
  - Pasty complexion
  - Elastic, nonpitting edema, particularly pretibially
  - Bradycardia, occasionally with syncope
  - Hypothermia
  - Pericardial effusions
- Laboratory findings:
  - T_3 and T_4 diminished
  - Hypercholesterolemia
  - Respiratory acidosis
  - Hyponatremia, hypokalemia
- *Differential diagnosis:*
  - Hypothyroid coma secondary to hypopituitarism

Definitive Treatment

- Intensive monitoring and intensive care
- L-T_4 (levothyroxine; does not take effect until at least 5 h have elapsed), 200–400 µg initially, then 50–200 µg/d via IV infusion pump
- Hydrocortisone, 100 mg initially, then 50 mg q.i.d.

Complications

- Pneumonia; cardiocirculatory and renal failure

Coma in Acute Adrenal Failure

Definition – Etiology

- Acute Addison's disease following chronic adrenal failure
- Hemorrhage and necrosis due to acquired clotting disorders, especially in septicemia

Clinical Signs – Diagnosis

- Clinical symptoms:
  - Colicky upper abdominal pain with vomiting and diarrhea
  - Hypothermia
  - Hypotension and tachycardia
  - Impairment of renal function
  - Typical brown pigmentation of skin, skin creases, and mucous membranes as a sign of prolonged adrenal failure
- Laboratory findings:
  - $Na\downarrow$, $K\uparrow$, $Cl\downarrow$, $Ca\uparrow$ in serum
  - $Hct\uparrow$, $MCV\downarrow$
  - Hypoglycemia, azotemia
  - Metabolic acidosis
  - Plasma cortisol

Therapy

- Overall input-output balancing and monitoring; liberal administration of fluids
- 9-α-fluorocortisone 0.05–0.1 mg q 24 h desoxycorticosterone acetate 1–2 mg IM
- Hydrocortisone 50–100 mg q.i.d.; 100 mg initially in severe cases
- Catecholamines to stabilize blood pressure initially in severe hypotension

Definition

- Deficiency of anterior-lobe pituitary hormones, resulting in clinically evident secondary adrenal failure, secondary hypothyroidism, and deficiency of gonadotrophic hormones

Etiology – Pathogenesis

- Usually the end stage of anterior-lobe pituitary failure
- Acute development in conditions involving:
  - Shock
  - Craniocephalic trauma
  - Postpartum ischemic necrosis (Sheehan's syndrome)
- Deficiency of ACTH (adrenocorticotrophic hormone) and TSH (thyroid-stimulating hormone) are the immediate causes of coma

Diagnosis

- Clinical evidence:
  - History
  - Hypothermia
  - Hypoventilation
  - Bradycardia
  - Hypoglycemia
  - Hypotension
  - Alabaster complexion with deficient pigmentation
  - Testicular atrophy
- Laboratory evidence:
  - Hyponatremia
  - Hypoglycemia
  - CO_2 retention, respiratory acidosis
  - Cortisol and STH (somatotropic hormone) diminished
  - T_3, T_4 and TSH diminished
- *Differential diagnosis:*
  - Primary hypothyroid coma
  - Anorexia mentalis
  - Primary adrenal cortical failure

Therapy

- Overall input-output balancing and monitoring
- Mechanical ventilation in case of marked hypercapnia

Hypopituitary Coma

- Medication:
  - Immediately:
    Hydrocortisone 200 mg IV initially, followed by 50–100 mg at 4 h intervals
    Tapering off to maintenance dosage of 25–50 mg/d
  - After 12–24 h: L-T_3 (liothyronine) 12.5 µg b.i.d. initially, then stepwise increase to 100 µg/d IV. Titrate to effect

  Remember:
  Hyperthermic treatment is contraindicated.

Complications

- Pneumonia, circulatory collapse, renal failure

Definition

- Irreversible loss of function of the central nervous system. This condition is equivalent to death of the individual, and must therefore be differentiated from reversible loss of CNS function.
- Dissociated cerebral death may be the end stage of therapy-resistant, progressive coma, or may develop following cardiac arrest with prolonged latency before cardiopulmonary resuscitation was initiated (extended anoxia).

Etiology – Pathogenesis

- Any intra- or extracerebral conditions that may give rise to coma and thus to end-stage coma are potential causes. Once initiated, brain damage due to such conditions may progress independently of the triggering mechanism, leading to irreversible loss of function. In any case, the cerebral reaction is the same, and the course is uniform.
  The most frequent causes of dissociated cerebral death are:
  - Cerebrocranial trauma
  - Intracerebral hemorrhage
  - Cardiocirculatory arrest

Diagnosis

- Diagnosis of dissociated cerebreal death is always based on:
  1. Clinical neurologic findings
  2. Electroencephalogram
  3. Further examination
- Guidelines for diagnosis are those provided by the German EEG Society for establishing the time of death:
  1. Clinical neurologic findings:
     a) Complete unconsciousness
     b) Cerebral areflexia, i.e.:
        - No response to acoustic stimuli
        - No reaction to visual stimuli
        - Absence of corneal reflex
        - No reaction of pupils to light
        - Absence of oculocephalic reflexes
        - Absence of oculovestibular reflexes
     c) Complete absence of spontaneous motor action
     d) Complete absence of spontaneous respiration
     Remember:
     Regulation of temperature and circulation may be intact, but spinal reflexes are irrelevant for diagnosis. Maximum dilation of the pupils is not necessarily present.

163

2. EEG: A flat EEG reflecting complete cessation of cerebral electrical activity is of key importance, and is essential for diagnosis. The EEG must be taken under prespecified standardized conditions.
3. Further examination:
   a) Specific assays for poisons. Poisoning may lead to reversible loss of cerebral function, and must be ruled out in every coma of uncertain origin. In this context, CAT scans may aid in differentiating cerebral edema from cerebral death; the brain appears homogeneously dense in the latter.
   b) A so-called "stop angiogram" demonstrating stagnation of injected contrast dye due to circulatory arrest in the blood vessels of the brain in cerebral death is no longer required; some authors reject it entirely. The main arguments against the procedure are potential damage to the vessels from angiography and the ethical objection that it has no therapeutic implications.
   c) Evoked potentials (i.e., elicited either acoustically or via other senses) yield results comparable to those obtained by EEG, but are technically more elaborate and require special experience.

Differential Diagnosis

- Both clinical and electroencephalographic criteria of dissociated cerebral death may be mimicked by reversible loss of CNS function in:
  - prolonged hypothermia, which always involves considerable reduction of metabolic processes;
  - poisoning by hypnotic drugs, which may lead to reversible cerebral defectiveness, including isoelectric EEG.

Confirmation of dissociated cerebral death justifies cessation of treatment, and is a prerequisite for removing organs for transplantation. The consequences of dissociated cerebral death must be explained carefully to both relatives and personnel.

Pathophysiology – Etiology

- The term brain edema refers to an augmentation of intracellular and/or interstitial fluid that leads to increased intracranial pressure and interferes with circulation in the brain. The result is local tissue hypoxia with clinical signs of unconsciousness and centrally caused systemic disorders of respiration, circulation, and temperature regulation. Treatment of brain edema therefore involves both procedures directed at specific problems and overall intensive care.
- Causes of brain edema are many and varied:
  - Craniocerebral trauma
  - Poisoning
  - Infectious diseases
  - Space-occupying lesions
  - Hemorrhage
  - Surgery
  - Recent cardiopulmonary resuscitation
  - Metabolic disorders, especially hepatic failure
  - Sunstroke
- Measures to counteract brain edema are indicated whenever central dysregulatory disorders appear likely in any of the conditions listed above, and become mandatory at the latest when clinical evidence of brain edema develops. For example: Following successful cardiopulmonary resuscitation, treatment as for brain edema should always be initiated.

Diagnosis – Monitoring

- Specific treatment of brain edema requires monitoring and observation at regular intervals to obtain baseline data and to document the course.
  1. Clinical and neurological findings:
     - State of consciousness and reflexes
     - Respiration
     - Circulation
     - Temperature
     - Central venous pressure
  2. Laboratory findings:
     - Electrolytes and blood sugar
     - Hematology (Hb, Hct, platelet count)
     - Clotting status
     - BUN
     - Urinalysis
  3. Spinal tap is indicated only in exceptional cases (e.g., if infection is suspected), since it carries a risk of herniation. Herniation may be present even without evidence of papilledema, which takes some time to develop.

4. Monitoring of input-output fluid balance
5. Specific procedures:
   a) EEG
   b) CAT scan (mandatory if available, and transportation reasonably feasible)
   c) Assessment of intracranial pressure by:
      – Intraventricular measurement
      – Epidural measurement

Remember:
Determination of intracerebral pressure is desirable, but lack of facilities for the procedure should not deter from *specific* treatment.

Therapy

• Basic intensive care:
  – Early initiation of endotracheal intubation and ventilation in the event of respiratory failure or unconsciousness; moderate hyperventilation (P_aCO_2 about 30 mmHg)
  – Maintenance of input-output fluid and electrolyte balance
  – Sufficient caloric alimentation
  – Positioning with elevated head or chest
• Basic treatment of brain edema:
  1. Furosemide in small doses at regular intervals (e.g., 20–40 mg q 4–6 h). CVP should be maintained at 0–5 cm H_2O; replacement of extracellular fluid by IV electrolyte drip when appropriate (to counteract risk of circulatory collapse due to hypovolemia and venous vasodilation). The effect on intracranial pressure lasts 0.5–2 h.
  2. Osmotherapy with 25% mannitol IV always requires monitoring of brain pressure (variable efficacy in different individuals, risk of rebound effect, risk of heavier intracranial hemorrhaging). Initial dose 1 g/kg bw; the effect lasts 0.5–12 h.
  3. Dexamethasone as follows:
     – Initially 100 mg IV (still controversial)
     – Days 1– 3:   8 mg q 2 h
     – Days 4– 6:   8 mg q 4 h
     – Days 7–10:   4 mg q 4 h
     – Days 11–12:   further tapering by lengthening intervals.

Recent studies indicate that steroids are effective in focal brain edema, but not in diffuse, generalized brain edema (differentiation by CAT scan).

- Specific therapy of brain edema:
  For several clinical conditions involving cerebral edema, specific medication may be considered, although its use is not generally established procedure:
  1. Calcium antagonists (e.g., nimodipine) in acute cerebral infarction
  2. Hemodilution (likewise in acute cerebral infarction) with hydroxyethyl starch (500–1000 mL 10% solution, depending on cardiopulmonary factors)
  3. Glycerol lowers CSF (cerebrospinal fluid) pressure in cerebral edema caused by ischemia; divergent views on its use
  4. Barbiturates for cerebral protection in hypoxic brain lesions (especially following cardiopulmonary resuscitation): IV infusion of thiopental, 20 mg/kg bw over 6 h, followed by phenobarbital 125 mg q 12 h for 24 h
- Anticonvulsant therapy in cerebral edema:
  1. Phenytoin (e.g., initial dose: 18 mg/kg in physiologic saline as IV drip [max. 50 mg/min]); maintenance dosage: 4–7 mg/kg daily as continuous IV drip. Serum levels to be monitored if possible (therapeutic range: 10–20 mg/L)
  2. Phenobarbital (e.g., 200 mg IV q 4–6 h, if possible, with monitoring of serum levels); therapeutic range 15–40 µg/mL
- Under certain conditions, extracorporeal drainage of CSF via ventricular catheter

Complications

- Sequelae of brain edema:
  - Hypoxic brain damage
  - Arrest of brain circulation
  - Irreversible impairment of function
- Potential hazards of treatment procedures:
  - Dehydration
  - Circulatory collapse
  - Metabolic disorders (electrolytes, glucose)
  - Bacterial infection

Remember:
Although the risk of bacterial infection is increased by administration of steroids to intensive-care patients, *prophylactic* administration of antibiotics is not appropriate.

Definition

- Grand-mal epileptic seizures are usually of brief duration, and most attacks that do not occur in an in-hospital setting will have subsided by the time a physician arrives.
- Status epilepticus denotes lengthier generalized convulsions that respond poorly to initial therapy or return shortly, and involve prolonged or increasing impairment of consciousness.

Etiology

- The most important causes of status epilepticus are:
  - Brain tumors
  - Cerebrocranial trauma
  - Cerebrovascular accidents
  - Discontinuation of anticonvulsive medication
  - Alcohol withdrawal
  - Meningoencephalitis
  - Residual damage (after disease, trauma or brain surgery)
  - Rare causes, e.g., cerebral hypoxia, metabolic disorders

Diagnosis

See Definition.

Therapy

- Diazepam 10 mg IV; repeat after 20–30 min if necessary. Takes effect in 1 min; effect lasts 15–20 min. If effect is inadequate:
- Phenytoin 250 mg IV, load with 10–15 mg/kg, up to 1 g; Further administration of phenytoin according to drug level in blood
- Phenobarbital 300 mg IV; repeat as needed after 20–30 min. Takes effect in 20 min; effect lasts 24–36 h
- Basic intensive therapy (with intubation and ventilation for respiratory failure in seizure state)

Complications

- Trauma related to sudden loss of consciousness and muscle contractions: lacerations, hematomas, fractures, bone displacements, intracranial bleeding (particularly subdural hematomas)
- Critical hypertension
- Hyperthermia
- Increase of intracranial pressure

Definition

Hemorrhage from cerebral arteries into the subarachnoid space

Etiology – Pathogenesis

- The origin remains obscure in 30% of cases.
- In descending order of incidence, this is followed by:
  - aneurysms of the circle of Willis;
  - mycotic aneurysms;
  - arteriovenous angiomas.
- Subarachnoid hemorrhage is caused by rupture of an aneurysm.
- Depending on the extent, subarachnoid bleeding may progress to parenchymal or intraventricular bleeding.

Diagnosis

- Symptoms: excruciating headaches, usually of sudden onset and often related to physical exertion; occasionally preceded by headache attacks
  Nausea and vomiting
- Neurologic findings:
  - Moderate to marked meningismus
  - Cranial nerve deficiencies due to pressure exerted by the aneurysm
  - All grades of impairment of consciousness, depending on severity of bleeding and intraparenchymal involvement
  - Hypertension, usually marked
  - ECG alterations resembling those in ischemic heart disease (and often mistaken for underlying cardiac disease)

The *Hunt and Hess* classification of clinical severity is generally accepted:

Grade I	Asymptomatic, or mild cephalgia and slightly stiff neck
Grade II	Moderate to severe cephalgia, meningismus, no neurologic deficiencies; cranial nerve deficiencies possible
Grade III	Clouded consciousness, confusion, minor neurologic deficiencies
Grade IV	Stupor, moderate to severe unilateral palsy, autonomic nervous disorders
Grade V	Deep coma, extensor posturing, severe autonomic nervous disorders

Subarachnoid Hemorrhage

Clinical Workup

- Typical clinical symptoms
- Confirmation of diagnosis by CAT scan
- Lumbar puncture unnecessary if history and CAT scan reveal clear-cut evidence; contraindicated in grades II–IV (Hunt and Hess)
- Angiography: in grades I and II (Hunt and Hess) or after diagnosis has been confirmed by CAT scan
- EEG: usually reveals overall changes of varying degree
- Transcranial Doppler echography for assessment of vascular spasms

Differential Diagnosis

- Acute cervical spine syndrome
- Acute migraine headaches
- Meningoencephalitides

Remember: The combination of coma of uncertain origin + arterial hypertension + ECG changes compatible with cardiac ischemia is suggestive of subarachnoid hemorrhage.

Therapy

- Surgical therapy depends on the patient's clinical condition.
  - Grade I and II (Hunt and Hess): angiographic verification of bleeding site; consideration of prompt surgery (referral to a neurosurgical unit)
  - Grade III: individualized therapy after consultation with neurosurgeon and neurologist
  - Grades IV and V: no early surgery and thus no angiography
- Symptomatic therapy:
  - Analgesia and sedation
  - Antihypertensive therapy (see guidelines in Critical Hypertension and Hypertensive Emergencies [p. 107])
  - No drugs that counteract hyperfibrinolysis, since evidence of usefulness not convincing
  - Calcium antagonists generally accepted for prevention of spasms, e.g., nimodipine 1–3 mg/h
  - Prevention of seizures
  - Treatment of brain edema (see guidelines, p. 165)

Complications

- Arterial spasms, particularly between days 4 and 12, evoking new neurologic deficiencies
- Recurrent hemorrhage (critical period between days 8 and 12)
- Hydrocephalus as a late sequela (after 2–4 weeks)
- Thromboembolism in the course of ICU treatment
- Lethality (40% within the first 2 months) still high

Prognosis

The prognosis is improved by early surgical intervention (i.e., within the first 48–72 h) in stages I and II (Hunt and Hess).

Patients with low-grade subarachnoid hemorrhage and no evidence of an aneurysm on first- or second-time angiography have a favorable prognosis. Their risk of renewed bleeding and arterial spasms is low.

Etiology – Pathogenesis

- The following sources of *upper* gastrointestinal hemorrhaging, listed in their order of incidence, are:
  - Duodenal ulcers
  - Gastric (ventricular) ulcers
  - Acute gastric lesions (erosive bleeding and stress ulcers)
  - Esophageal varices
  - Mallory-Weiss lesions
  - Esophagitis
- Intensive monitoring is indicated in the event of:
  - Blood loss of more than 500–600 mL in 12 h
  - Tachycardia and drop in blood pressure, restlessness, clouding of consciousness, or manifest shock
- The most common sources of hemorrhage in the ICU are gastroduodenal stress ulceration and diffuse bleeding from that region in conjunction with severe clotting disorders.

Diagnosis

- Hematemesis, tarry or bloody stools
- Signs of hypovolemia
  Remember:
  Impairment of GI-tract motility may permit undetected sequestration of large amounts of blood. Hypovolemic shock may be the initial symptom under such conditions.
- Recovery of blood via gastric tube, which should be inserted early for diagnostic purposes
- Emergency endoscopy indicated for verification of source of bleeding in all cases of active, severe hemorrhage
- Estimation of severity of bleeding from amounts of blood passed and from serial assessments of CVP, BP (blood pressure), and Hb

Immediate Care

- A central venous line should be established and an immediate blood sample drawn for:
  - Hematology
  - Electrolyte assessment
  - Quick's test, PTT, TT (thrombin time), and platelet count
  - BUN
  - Blood crossmatching
- Large-bore peripheral IV line for volume replacement and blood transfusion

- Infusion of plasma extenders, depending on blood pressure, heart-rate (HR), and CVP: $CVP \geq 4\,cm\;H_2O$, $HR < 90/min$, systolic arterial $BP > 100\,mmHg$
- Nasogastric tube
- Rinsing of the stomach to clarity
- Endotracheal intubation in the event of clouding of consciousness or overt shock to prevent aspiration
- Once the patient's condition is stable, endoscopic (in exceptional cases, angiographic) verification of the source of bleeding

Continuing Care

- Variceal hemorrhage:
1. Vasopressin infusion: Start at 0.2–0.4 U/min; up to 1.0 U/min may be needed. Vasopressin may be administered in an emergency or as trial of treatment before insertion of a Sengstaken-Blakemore tube or Linton-Nachlas tube. If bleeding persists after 2–4 h, balloon tamponade or injection of sclerosing solution is appropriate.
2. Balloon tamponade with:
   a) Sengstaken-Blakemore tube (double-balloon, 3-lumen):
      - Introduce through the nose.
      - Inflate the gastric balloon with 200 cc of air→Retract, and weight down with 250 g across a pulley→Inflate the esophageal balloon with 100 cc of air, adjust pressure to starting level of 40–50 mmHg→Mark initial position of the tube→Verify position by x-ray.
   b) Linton-Nachlas tube (single balloon, 3 lumens) is primarily suited for fundal varices.
      - Introduce as for Sengstaken-Blakemore tube.
      - Fill balloon with 600 cc of air→Weight down pulley with 1000 g→Mark position of the tube→Verify position by x-ray.
   Remember:
   Constant monitoring is required: Pressure checks of the esophageal balloon in the Sengstaken-Blakemore tube at regular intervals, rinsing of stomach to empty it, aspiration of pharyngeal contents, checks of position of the tube.
3. Sclerosing injections:
   Indications are varied:
   - Following successful balloon tamponade
   - If bleeding persists despite balloon tamponade
   - As first-line hemostyptic procedure, possibly after an emergency vasopressin drip
4. In all cases cessation of bleeding should be followed by cleansing and antibiotic clearing of the intestine.

Upper Gastrointestinal Hemorrhage

- Hemorrhage from ulcers and erosive lesions:
  1. *Local treatment:* Rinse to clear at regular intervals. After bleeding has stopped, antacids may be instilled (at the earliest after 24 h). Local application of hemostatic agents has little merit and is not very effective.
  2. *Systemic medication:*
     a) Hemostasis:
        - Somatostatin 250 μg bolus IV, followed by 250 μg/h as continuous IV drip
     b) Facilitation of healing and prevention of further hemorrhage: Ranitidine (H_2-receptor blocker): 50 mg q 4–6 h, provided renal function is normal. Dosage must be adjusted if renal function is impaired.
        Remember: H_2-receptor blockers may cause a decrement of WBCs and platelets (reversible on discontinuation); impairment of consciousness occurs rarely.
  3. Endoscopic therapy depends on the local situation:
     - Injection deep to the bleeding site, or sclerosis
     - Laser coagulation
  4. Surgical intervention in event of:
     - Arterial spurting
     - Visible vascular pedicle on endoscopy
     - Transfusion of more than 4–6 units of blood in 24 h

- Prevention of stress bleeding:
  - Appropriate treatment of predisposing conditions, particularly shock, clotting disorders, hypercatabolism, and renal or respiratory failure
  - Antacids, preferably with pH monitoring of gastric juices (pH should exceed 3.5) q 4 h: aspiration of gastric juice, dipstick assessment of pH. If pH < 3.5, antacid dosage should be doubled; if it is > 3.5, the dosage should be maintained.
    If pH checks are not feasible: administration of a Mg-Al compound in 30 mL H_2O q 4 h.
  - H_2-receptor blocking agents should be used judiciously for prevention. Unreflected administration to every patient in the ICU is contraindicated. GI flora may be altered following pH changes of gastric juice; this should be considered in conjunction with the hazard of aspiration of microorganisms, and is conducive to nosocomial pneumonias.
    Remember:
    Optimum sedation (in which the patient responds only when spoken to directly or touched, while tolerating all other intensive care procedures) serves well to prevent stress ulcers.

Complications

- Overt shock with respiratory and renal failure
- Clotting disorders (massive transfusion)
- Aspiration (especially when balloon tamponade is in situ)
- Pressure necrosis due to balloon tamponade

Definition

Autodigestive, tryptic pancreatitis, the hemorrhagic-necrotizing form of which gives rise to reactive circulatory impairment and to complications involving other organs

Etiology – Pathogenesis

- The most frequent underlying causes of pancreatitis are:
  - Biliary tract disease
  - Alcoholism
- The key event in pathogenesis that determines the extent and severity of clinical symptoms is proteolytic autodigestion of the organ:

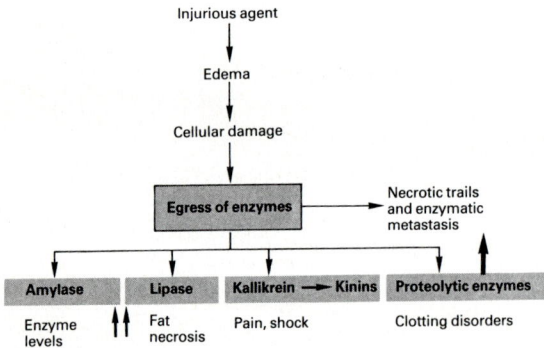

Diagnosis

- Symptoms and signs:
  1. Chief clinical symptom is *abdominal pain* accompanied by:
     - Nausea, vomiting
     - Tympanitic distension of the abdomen, starting in the upper abdomen, with typical muscular defense (so-called rubber belly)
     - Subileus, Ileus
     - Symptoms of shock
  2. Organ complications:
     - Acute renal failure
     - Acute respiratory failure
     - Left-sided pleural effusions containing enzymes
     - Disseminated intravascular clotting
     - Gastrointestinal bleeding

3. Laboratory findings:
   - Leukocytosis
   - Elevated α-amylase levels in serum and urine (decreasing after 2–3 days if necrosis is widespread)
   - Elevated serum lipase levels (hyperlipasemia persists longer than hyperamylasemia, but both enzymes may be undetectable following total pancreatic necrosis)
   - Diminished serum calcium levels (levels below 1.5 mmol/L are indicative of a severe course)
   - Hyperglycemia
   - Metabolic acidosis
   - Hyperlactatemia
   - Electrolyte derangements
   - In severe cases: signs of the organ complications listed above
4. Other findings and diagnostic procedure:
   - Abdominal girth, abdominocentesis (ascites fluid contains enzymes)
   - Plain abdominal x-rays
   - Ultrasound
   - CAT scan

   Remember:
   Due to its aggressive course and rapid progression, acute pancreatitis requires frequent monitoring of all aforementioned parameters. Repeated, collaborative examination by internists and surgeons is recommended.

- Degrees of severity:

1st stage (edematous pancreatitis)	– Moderate tenderness – Markedly enhanced enzyme levels – No electrolyte disorders, no acidosis – Good response to conservative treatment
2nd stage (partially necrotizing pancreatitis)	– Marked abdominal tenderness with muscular defense and pathologic rigidity due to necrotic trails – Enzyme levels moderately enhanced – Moderate hypocalcemia, acidosis, and hyperlactacidema – Moderate response to basic conservative treatment
3rd stage (total pancreatic necrosis)	– Massive abdominal pathology (rubber belly) – Enzymes moderately elevated or normal – Marked biochemical pathology with involvement of other organs – No response to conservative treatment measures

- *Differential diagnosis:*
  Any condition involving acute abdomen:
  - Acute inflammation of intraabdominal organs
  - Perforating ulcer
  - Intestinal obstruction
  - Occlusion of mesenteric vein or artery
  - GI bleeding
  - Intraabdominal bleeding

Therapy

- Intensive therapy:
  - Basic therapy: avoidance of demands on pancreatic function, and prevention or early treatment of complications in other organs
  - Sedation, analgesia
  - Gastric tube with suction drainage
  - Fasting diet with adequate parenteral caloric intake
  - Input-output balancing of electrolytes, fluids, and acid-base status (fluid requirements are rarely below 2.5–3.5 L/d)
  - Replacement of lost protein
  - Treatment of shock
  - Prophylactic administration of heparin
  - Prompt administration of antibiotics
  - Prompt initiation of appropriate treatment of complications involving other organs:
    1. Prompt initiation of dialysis in acute renal failure (see p. 125)
    2. Prompt initiation of PEEP ventilation in respiratory failure
- Evaluation of specific drugs:
  - Atropine:
    In dosages that inhibit secretion, specific side effects predominate. Atropine should not be given.
  - Calcitonin:
    alleviates symptoms, especially pain, but not the course. It may mask the severity of the condition. Final evaluation is not yet possible. Dosage: 300 IU/24 h.
  - Glucagon:
    fails to exert a favorable effect on the course.
  - Somatostatin:
    Experience is limited, due to multicentric design of studies. Dosage: 250 µg as IV bolus, then 250 µg/h as IV drip.
  - H_2-receptor blocking agents:
    seem logical because they inhibit of excessive production of gastric secretion.

- Medical vs. surgical treatment:
  - 1st- and 1st/2nd stage pancreatitis: conservative therapy
  - 2nd degree pancreatitis: An expectant attitude and intensive care are justified in the absence of complications in other organs and as long as abdominal findings do not deteriorate; surgery (left-sided resection) after stabilization in the postacute phase
  - 3rd stage pancreatitis: prompt surgery (necrosectomy or left-sided resection), i.e., before organ complications become resistant to treatment. Reason: The course is lethal in total necrosis of the pancreas with overt complications in other organs.
  - Postsurgical continuation of intensive care (see above), especially postoperative PEEP ventilation until pulmonary function is stable
- Peritoneal lavage
  Reports differ, but some indicate very positive results by various teams, both in 2nd- and 3rd-stage pancreatitis.

Complications

- Functional impairment of other organs (see above)
- Diffuse purulent peritonitis
- Intraabdominal abscess formation following temporary improvement

Prognosis

- Depends on degree of severity. Lethality of edematous pancreatitis is practically zero, that of total necrosis with organ complications is nearly 100%. Lethality data are therefore subject to interpretation only in relation to stage of severity.
- Intensive care and prompt surgical intervention have lowered the lethality even of hemorrhagic-necrotizing pancreatitis. The greatest improvement has been achieved in partial necrosis of the pancreas, but individual cases of recovery have been reported for total necrosis as well.

Bowel Obstruction and Peritonitis

Etiology – Pathophysiology

- Mechanical strangulation or obstruction of the bowel
- Paralytic (adynamic) ileus with peritonitis in the following disorders:
  - Intra- and retroperitoneal bacterial or abacterial inflammations
  - Pancreatic and biliary disorders
  - Occlusion of mesenteric artery or vein
  - GI bleeding
  - Diabetic, hepatic, or uremic coma
  - Acute intermittent porphyria
  - Acute peroral intoxication
  - Postsurgical ileus
- Self-perpetuating complications:
  - Shock (hypovolemic and/or septic)
  - Acute renal impairment with risk of acute renal failure
  - Acute respiratory impairment with risk of ARDS

Diagnosis

- Depends on type and severity of the basic condition and on the extent of peritoneal reaction:
  1. Mechanical ileus:
     - Crampy pain and persistent intestinal contraction proximal to the obstruction
     - Depending on the location of the blockage, early reflexive vomiting (proximal lesion) or early retention of stools and flatulence (distal lesion)
     - Bowel sounds increased, tinkling, high-pitched
     - Tympanitic abdominal distension
  2. Paralytic ileus:
     - Retention of flatulence and stools
     - Absence of intestinal sounds
     - Vomiting
     - Tympanitic abdominal distension
  3. Acute peritonitis:
     - Boardlike abdominal rigidity
     - Peritoneal pain (tenderness, pain on percussion, rebound pain)
     - Absence of bowel sounds
     - Vomiting
     - Superficial, rapid respiration
     - Cold sweating
     - Rapid onset of shock symptoms

- Laboratory diagnosis:
  a) Parameters of the basic protocol (see p. 21), plus serum amylase and lipase
  b) Specific tests that may reveal etiology and indicate severity of the course:
    - Blood cultures (aerobic and anaerobic) and bacteriology of drainage tubes, fistulas, and ascites fluid
    - Serum lactic acid
    - Quantitative urinalysis
    - δ-Aminolevulinic acid and porphobilinogen in urine
- Other diagnostic procedures:
  - Plain abdominal x-rays
  - Echography
  - CAT scan
  - Water-soluble contrast x-rays without barium for identification and localization of intestinal obstruction
  - Angiography if specifically indicated
  - Emergency laparoscopy and exploratory laparotomy if the cause cannot be identified by other means
- *Differential diagnosis:*
  Disorders requiring immediate surgical intervention must be ruled out.
  1. Surgical conditions:
     - Mechanical ileus
     - Appendicitis
     - Intraabdominal abscesses and emphysemas
     - Perforations
     - Intraabdominal hemorrhage
  2. Medical conditions:
     - Metabolic disorders (e.g., diabetes, porphyria)
     - Primary bacterial peritonitis (very rare)
     - Pancreatitis stages I–II (see p. 177)
  Remember:
  Diagnosis and differentiation are particularly difficult in patients undergoing mechanical ventilation, sedation, or muscular relaxation. Useful triad for identification of sepsis:
  - Decrement in platelet count
  - Hypophosphatemia
  - Leucocytosis with leftward shift

Bowel Obstruction and Peritonitis

Intensive Care

- Indwelling nasogastric tube, not clamped off, preferably with constant suction (see p. 16)
- Maintenance of vital functions:
  - Accurate input-output balancing and replacement of protein, fluid, and electrolytes, and correction of acid-base imbalance
  - Parenteral alimentation
  - Antibiotics
  - Prophylactic administration of heparin (see p. 302)
  - Early initiation of ventilation
  - Early initiation of hemodialysis
  - Measures to counteract shock
  - Sympathicolysis with chlorpromazine and dihydroergotamine and/or parasympathetic stimulation (e.g., neostigmine)
- Prompt surgical intervention for the diagnoses listed above as "surgical"; postoperative intensive care

Complications

- Septicemia with septic shock and metabolic coma
- Organ complications: acute renal impairment, acute respiratory failure, GI bleeding
- Disseminated intravascular clotting (see page 183)

Prognosis

- Depends on extent of compromise of vital functions
- Particularly poor if sepsis develops
- Lethality is 100% in peritonitis requiring dialysis for acute renal failure and mechanical ventilation for respiratory failure, if the peritonitis cannot be treated by surgery ("lethal triad")

Disseminated Intravascular Coagulation (DIC)

Definition

- Typical acquired clotting disorders in ICU patients are disruption of the normal balance between latent clotting and latent fibrinolysis by activation of one or the other or both systems:
  - Disseminated intravascular coagulation (DIC)
  - Hyperfibrinolysis
- Combinations and gradual transition of the two disorders may occur.

Etiology – Pathogenesis

- Accelerated intravascular turnover of plasma clotting factors with inadequate reactive augmentation of fibrinolysis:
  - This leads to thrombotic occlusions in the microcirculation→cellular death→organ death.
  - Hemorrhagic diathesis develops either simultaneously or somewhat later, caused by rapid consumption of clotting factors.

Remember:
DIC should be considered whenever bleeding occurs in conjunction with organ failure.

- Causes:
  1. Endogenous:
     - Shock
     - Bacteria, viruses, and bacterial endotoxins
     - Hemolysis
     - Hemorrhagic necrosis of the pancreas
     - Liver disease

     Remember:
     Differentiation between disorders of synthesis and DIC in hepatic disorders may be difficult. The most important criterion is factor VIII, which is synthesized outside the liver.
     - Absorbed poisons
     - Massive transfusions
     - Acidosis

     Remember:
     Metabolic acidosis may either cause DIC, or develop consequent upon it.
  2. Exogenous, consequent upon:
     - Trauma
     - Thermic burns
     - Chemical burns
     - Amniotic fluid embolism
     - Surgical procedures on the uterus, lungs, or prostate (risk of releasing active clotting factors)
     - Abruptio placentae
     - Malignant tumors

Disseminated Intravascular Coagulation (DIC)

Diagnosis

- The most important clinical symptom are profuse cutaneous and mucocutaneous bleeding and necrosis, accompanied by organ failure. The organs most frequently affected and the symptoms they produce with or without bleeding are:
  - Lungs: Respiratory failure
  - Kidneys: Oligoanuria
  - Skin: Necrosis
  - Circulation: Shock
  - GI tract: Ileus
  - Adrenals: Failure
  - Joint and muscles: Hemorrhaging

  Remember:
  Clinical symptoms are always late signs of increased turnover and signalize overt DIC.

- *Clotting Status:*
  - Platelet count below 50,000/mm^3, or rapid drop from normal levels within a period of hours
  - PTT markedly prolonged
  - Prothrombin time markedly prolonged (Quick's test below 40%)
  - Reptilase time or thrombin coagulase time somewhat prolonged or normal
  - Fibrinogen normal or somewhat diminished
  - Evidence of fibrin monomers and fibrin(ogen) split products
  - Factors V, VIII, IX, X, XII, and XIII markedly diminished
  - Diminished level of AT (antithrombin) III
  - Drop in plasma prekallikrein
  - Remember:
    Essential for diagnosis and monitoring: PTT, TT, reptilase time of thrombin coagulase time, Quick's test, platelet count
    Desirable, if available: fibrin(ogen) split-product titer, AT III, plasma prekallikrein

- Laboratory evidence of organ impairment:
  - Rising creatinine levels
  - Increasing transaminase activity
  - Increasing levels of amylase and lipase

- *Differential diagnosis:*
  - Congenital coagulopathy
  - Thrombocytopenia of other origin and thrombocytopathias
  - Vascular and capillary damage
  - Pure synthesis disorders
  - Primary hyperfibrinolysis (see below)

Intensive Therapy

- Elimination of causative factors
- Heparin 500–1000 IU/h, preferably as continuous IV drip, to interrupt the coagulation process
- Frequent monitoring for evaluation of therapy and identification of secondary hyperfibrinolysis
  Remember:
  When clotting factors are replaced by *blood components,* heparin must also be given to prevent further activation of the coagulation process. If heparin is ineffective in arresting consumption, deficiency of AT III is the most frequent reason. AT III may be given in concentrated form or as fresh plasma.
- Drug-induced thrombolysis may be considered as a last-resort procedure in fulminant courses.

Complications

- Organ complications due to microthrombosis and/or hemorrhage
- Hemorrhage due to overdosage of heparin
  Remember:
  The appropriate dosage of heparin must be titrated to fit individual needs, especially if there is renal impairment (with bleeding tendency)
- Heparin-specific side effects

Prognosis

- The prognosis depends largely on eliciting factors and the underlying condition.
- Prompt initiation of heparin therapy is as important as expeditious elimination of causes of DIC, which are usually multiple.
- The prognosis also depends on how well the specific therapy is integrated in general intensive therapy or organ complications:
  - Early initiation of mechanical ventilation
  - Treatment of acute renal failure by early initiation of hemodialysis

Follow-up Treatment

- Administration of heparin until:
  - clotting factors have returned to normal levels;
  - bleeding has ceased;
  - eliciting factors have been eliminated.

Etiology – Pathogenesis

- Plasmin is the active proteolytic enzyme of the fibrinolysis system. Sudden, overshooting fibrinokinase activity gives rise to plasmin concentrations that can no longer be kept in check by natural plasmin inhibitors, resulting in hyperfibrinolysis.
  1. *Primary hyperfibrinolysis* is a potential threat in disorders of organs with high fibrinokinase activity, e.g., uterus, lungs, prostate, and lymph nodes:
     - Aspiration of amniotic fluid
     - Retroplacental hematoma
     - Intestinal bleeding
     - Hepatic cirrhosis
     - Leukemia
     Primary hyperfibrinolysis accounts for no more than 1% of all hemorrhaging not due to mechanical factors.
  2. *Secondary hyperfibrinolysis*. The most common overall cause of fibrinolysis is DIC. DIC in turn elicits reactive fibrinolysis, which may partially or wholly compensate the DIC. Hyperfibrinolysis may be so overwhelming that it dominates the entire clinical picture.

Diagnosis

- Chief symptom is sudden onset of massive hemorrhage.
- Analysis of clotting factors shows the following deviations from findings in DIC:
  - Fibrinogen markedly diminished
  - Thrombin time significantly prolonged
  - Reptilase time significantly prolonged
  - Only slight platelet depletion
  - Fibrin split products markedly enhanced
  - Plasminogen diminished

Intensive Therapy

- Causative factors must be eliminated. Attention must never be directed to coagulation therapy alone.
- ε-aminocaproic acid (Amicar) may be used; Loading dose of 4–5 g is followed by an IV infusion at 1 g/h until bleeding subsides.
  In *secondary hyperfibrinolysis:*
  - Caution must be exercised to avoid premature administration of antifibrinolytic agents

- Antifibrinolytic agents should not be given unless levels of coagulation factors in plasma fail to increase, and deficiency of AT III is ruled out as the cause thereof, or excessive fibrinolytic activity has been verified.

Remember:

Differentiation may be difficult. Monitoring of the following coagulation factors *at least* q 6–8 h is essential:

- Thrombin time
- Prothrombin time
- Reptilase time
- Fibrinogen level
- Quick's test
- Platelet count
- Fibrin split-products titer, if available

Subsequent Therapy

- Heparin in preventive dosage
- Cautious replacement of clotting factors
- Transfusion of fresh blood only, if possible

Complications

- Thrombosis and microthrombosis if antifibrinolytic therapy is initiated too early or not indicated
- Organ complications as in DIC, further complicated by hemorrhaging

Prognosis

- Due to the fulminant course with life-threatening blood loss, generally worse than in DIC, and more difficult to treat

Definition

- Simultaneous or rapidly consecutive failure of 2 or more vital organs. Typical manifestations in organ systems are acute respiratory failure, acute renal failure, acute gastrointestinal lesions, acute hepatic failure, metabolic decompensation, and clotting disorders.

Etiology – Pathogenesis

- Medical patients at risk for multiorgan failure are those with severe poisoning, severe pneumonia, severe CNS infections, or upper abdominal disease (particularly pancreatitis).
  Surgical patients at risk are those with polytrauma, major surgery, severe abdominal disorders, and complications.

- Septicemia is one of the main pathogenetic factors in multiorgan failure, but the latter may also occur in nonsepticemic patients (e.g., following polytrauma or poisoning, or in pancreatitis). Other pathogenetic links between the underlying disorder and multiorgan failure are shock and DIC.

- Temporal sequence: Acute respiratory failure usually develops first; after a few days it is followed by acute hepatic failure, stress bleeding, and acute renal failure.

Diagnosis

- The diagnosis is based on failure of 2 or more of the aforementioned organ systems in a critically ill patient. The usual criteria for diagnosis of failure of each organ retain their validity.

Intensive Therapy

- In therapy, the rules for treating disorders of each organ system apply.
- Due to the unfavorable prognosis in overt multiorgan failure, prompt initiation of precise intensive monitoring and intensive care are required for early identification and treatment of organ failure, or – if possible – to prevent it from becoming manifest at all.

Prognosis

- Lethality of overt multiple organ failure is 60–80%. It increases with the number of organ systems simultaneously affected; in case of acute respiratory failure requiring mechanical ventilation and acute renal failure requiring dialysis, the lethality is 90%.

- Exogenous poisoning accounts for 5–10% of all admissions to medical departments, which is about equivalent to the quota for myocardial infarction. About 15–20% of emergency ambulance calls are for poisoning. In medical ICUs, 20–40% of the patients are treated for poisoning.
  Intoxications are the most frequent cause of nontraumatic coma in adults (35–40% of all nontraumatic comas).

- Causes of poisoning:
  80–90% of intoxication cases among adults involve intentional intake of poison for suicidal purposes, 10–15% are accidental, and about 5% occupation-related.

- Types of poisons:
  – Medicines are involved in 80–90% of all poisoning cases, making them the most frequent cause. Hypnotic and psychotropic drugs, mostly tranquilizers, predominate with 85%, of these ⅓–⅔ being psychotropic agents, and ½–⅔ hypnotic drugs. In the latter group, the frequency of barbiturate poisoning has decreased in favor of a higher incidence of poisoning by nonbarbiturate sleep-inducing drugs. Analgesics account for about 5%.
  Remember:
  If only *extremely severe* cases are considered, barbiturates still account for the greatest portion.
  – Categorization may be difficult, for poisoning with a combination of several different agents is involved in at least half of the cases. Toxicological analysis permits identification only of the major components. The combination of medication with toxic amounts of alcohol is seen much more frequently than severe intoxication with alcohol alone.

- Distribution according to sex: ratio of females to males 2:1, due to the higher frequency of suicidal poisonings in women

- Age profile: peak frequency in the 20- to 40-year age group

- The following sections deal with general procedures in patients with exogenous poisoning. Specialized literature must be consulted regarding poisoning by individual substances.

- Goals of treatment in exogenous intoxication:
  – Overcoming or prevention of life-threatening disorders that result directly from effects of the poison or from complications secondary to it
  – Prevention or treatment of organ damage due to effects of the poison

- Basic therapy consists of:
  - *General basic therapy:* basic emergency treatment and intensive care procedures to restore and maintain vital functions.
  - *Specific detoxification therapy:* specific emergency and intensive care procedures to remove or neutralize poison that may not yet have been absorbed, counteract toxic effects, and accelerate excretion of poison that may already have been absorbed

Outside of hospital:

- Inspection of the patient's surroundings for empty drug packages, bottles, or glasses with suspicious contents
- Questioning of the patient and contact persons: What? When? How? How much? Why? Remarks expressing lack of will to live or suicidal intent?
- Common symptoms of poisoning:
  1. CNS disorders:
     - CNS depression with impaired consciousness or coma
     - CNS excitation with restlessness, confusion, excitation, agitation, tremor, seizures
  2. Gastrointestinal symptoms:
     Nausea, retching, vomiting, diarrhea
  3. Dermal lesions:
     - Erythema, followed by blisters with central necrosis may develop in unconscious patients lying down for lengthy periods (i.e., more than 6–8 h) following poisoning by hypnotic or psychotropic drugs (so-called barbiturate blisters); vulnerable sites: ankles, knees, hips, shoulders
     - Chemical burns following ingestion of corrosive substances
     - Burn-like skin alterations after contact with solvents and other chemicals
     - Remarkable odor
       (Odor of breath or vomitus may suggest type of poisoning.)
- Telephone information from regional Poison Control Centers.

On Admission

- Toxicologic screening:
  - Toxicologic screening tests (see Table **12**)
  - Gas detector: instrumental identification of gases or vapors, particularly in exhaled air or in vomitus
  - Plain abdominal films to reveal masses of bromide sleeping pills in the stomach
  - Screening tests in the event of medicinal poisoning (enzyme or radioimmunoassays, thin-layer chromatography)
- Laboratory findings:
  Marked enhancement of CK activity in serum of unconscious patients who lack signs of trauma or intracranial hemorrhage
- Toxicologic proof of poison in stomach contents, urine, or blood (serum)

Table **12**   Toxicologic screening tests

Substance Category	Test	Reaction
Barbiturates	Chloroform extract + cobalt acetate + lithium hydroxide	Turns light blue
Phenothiazine	FPN reagent	Turns orange-violet
Paraquat, deiquat	Alkalinization + sodium thionate	Turns blue-green
Organic phosphates	Cholinesterase	Inhibition of activity

- Life-saving emergency procedures:
  The basic rules for all emergencies are also valid for poisoning:
  - Lateral recumbent positioning
  - Clearing of airways and keeping them open
  - Mechanical ventilation in case of respiratory failure or apnea
  - Cardiopulmonary resuscitation in the event of cardiocirculatory arrest
  - IV infusions and volume replacement in the event of shock
  Disorders of vital functions common in poisoning:
  - Unconsciousness
  - Impairment of respiratory function (respiratory paralysis, airways obstruction, aspiration, bronchial tree obstruction, disorders of O_2 transportation)
  - Cardiocirculatory disorders (shock, cardiocirculatory arrest, heart failure, cardiac arrythmias)
- Rescue:
  In poisoning by inhalation of toxic fumes or gases, the victim must be evacuated from the contaminated area.
- Skin cleansing:
  In case of potential transcutaneous penetration of the poison, remove contaminated clothing and cleanse the skin thoroughly.
- Induction of vomiting:
  1. Indication: highly suspected or verified ingestion of toxic substances by alert, cooperative patients
  2. Contraindications:
     - Impaired consciousness or unconsciousness, due to possibility of aspiration (alternative: gastric lavage)
     - Ingestion of corrosive substances, due to risk of damage to esophagus and larynx by regurgitation (alternative: dilution by having patient drink large amounts of water)
     - Ingestion of frothing substances, due to risk of respiratory impairment (alternative: administration of foam inhibitors)
     - Ingestion of organic solvents, due to risk of severe lung damage (alternative: activated charcoal; see p. 195)
  3. Induction of emesis by saline:
     - 1–2 glases of warm, hypertonic saline (2 tbsp. salt per glass water) drunk rapidly
     - In the event of retching without vomiting, patient to drink plenty of water or juice to induce copious vomiting
     - Further provocation or intensification of reflexive emesis by mechanical stimulation of the pharynx
     - Applicable in adults and children above the age of 10–12 years
     Remember:
     If hypertonic saline fails to induce emesis, the stomach must be evacuated via tube and gastric lavage to prevent salt poisoning from absorption of large amounts of NaCl.

4. Technique of inducing emesis by ipecac syrup:
   – Administration of ipecac syrup: children under 1.5 years, 10 mL; children from 1.5 to 12 years, 15 mL; children over 12 years, 30 mL, followed by:
   – Administration of fluid (juice, tea, water) by mouth; vomiting should ensue within 20 min
   – In appropriate cases, stimulation of the pharynx to provoke or enhance vomiting
   – Contraindicated in children under 8 months of age
- Neutralization of poisons:
1. Ingestion of corrosive substances:
   – Dilution at effective site by having patient drink large amounts of fluid (tea, juice, or water)
   – Administration of antacids in case of acidic poisoning
   – Administration of diluted vinegar (1% = 3 tbsp. household vinegar in 1 glass water) or lemon juice in case of poisoning by alkaline substances
2. Ingestion of frothing substances:
   – Administration of antifoaming agents, e.g., simethicone
3. Ingestion of oily solutions or organic solvents:
   – Activated charcoal; in severe poisoning, 30 g via gastric tube
   Activated charcoal is always appropriate, except in cases of ingestion of acids or alkalis. The largest possible dose should be given: in severe cases, 30 g in suspension via gastric tube.
- Antidotes (see Table **13**):
Emergency measures that may be performed away from hospital facilities in severe cases where basic procedures are insufficient. Antidotes should be given *outside the hospital* only for:
1. Ingestion of "organophosphates:"
   – Atropine 1–2 mg IV initially, followed by 0.5–2 mg, depending on bronchial secretion and hypersalivation
2. Cyanide poisoning:
   – Amyl nitrite 1 ampoule to be inhaled by the patient, if sodium nitrite is not available
   – Sodium nitrite 6.6 mg/kg initially, *then* 50 ml/kg of 25% solution sodium thiosulfate slowly IV (enhances formation of ferrihemoglobin, and has fewer side effects than nitrites)
   Sodium thiosulfate *after* administration of DMAP, 50–100 mg/kg slowly IV
3. Methanol poisoning:
   – Ethanol by mouth (about 100 mL 50% liquor, e.g., whisky)
   – Ethanol IV drip, to achieve blood alcohol levels around 0.001 mg/dL

Table **13**   Antidotes for treatment of poisoning

Indication	Antidote	Dosage
1. Alkylated phosphates	Atropine	Initiate with 1–2 mg within 15 min, then IV drip at 0.5–2 mg/h
2. Barium	Sodium sulfate	15 g orally (2 g for each g $BaCl_2$)
3. Lead	Calcium disodium edetate	Initiate with 15–20 mg/kg IV drip over a 2-h period; long-term treatment up to 50 mg/kg daily
4. Cyanide	Sodium thiosulfate	Initiate with sodium nitrite 6.6 mg/kg, then 50 ml/kg of 25% solution
5. Digitalis	Digoxin immune Fab (Digibind, Burroughs-Wellcome)	Adjust dosage in accordance with serum concentrations: 80 mg antitoxin will inactivate 1 mg digitalis (5–20 vialo)
6. Dextro-propoxyphene	Naloxone	0.01 mg/kg IV, maximum 8 times; 0.1 mg/kg may be needed for severe poisoning
7. Iron	Deferoxamine mesylate	1–2 g parenterally
8. Gold	Dimercaprol	1–4 g orally daily
9. INH	Vitamin B6	20 mg/100 mg INH IM or by mouth
10. Methadone	Naloxone	0.01 mg/kg IV; repeat up to 8 times
11. Neuroleptic drugs	Biperiden	0.04 mg/kg slowly IV or IM; repeat up to 4 times
	Diphenhydramine HCl	50 mg IV slowly, or IM
12. Opiates	Naloxone	0.01 mg/kg IV (up to 0.1 mg/kg); repeat up to 8 times
13. Acetamino-phen	N-acetylcysteine	Initiate with 140 mg/kg, then 70 mg/kg q 4 h, for 17 doses (68 h)
14. Mercury (inorganic)	Dimercaprol (BAL in oil)	5 mg/kg IM
15. Toxic fumes	Dexamethasone	Initiate with 2–4 sprays, then 2 sprays q 10 min until contents are used up
16. Anti-cholinergic syndrome	Physostigmine sulfate	Initial dose (2 mg) takes effect in 5–10 min; effect lasts 20 min to hours; repeat if necessary

4. Narcotic poisoning:
   - In threatened or actual respiratory paralysis without facilities for intubation: naloxone 0.01 mg/kg IV (0.1 mg/kg may be needed); repeat up to 8 times
5. Inhalation of toxic fumes:
   - Steroids in metered aerosolized canisters, to be inhaled by the victim: initially, 2–4 sprays of dexamethasone, followed by 2 sprays at 10-min intervals until the container is empty

- *Primary detoxification* for removal of poisons before they are absorbed:
1. Cleanse skin thoroughly (see p. 193).
2. Induce vomiting (see p. 193).
3. Insert gastric tube; gastric lavage:
   a) Indications:
      - Marked clouding of consciousness or unconsciousness in cases of suspected or verified peroral poisoning
      - Always indicated after ingestion of highly toxic substances, e.g., organic phosphates, deiquat or paraquat, or heavy metals, even if the patient has vomited
      - If attempts to induce emesis with hypertonic saline fail
   b) Prerequisites:
      Feasibility of endotracheal intubation and consideration of the indications for intubation before performing gastric lavage:
      - Protective pharyngeal reflexes (choking, swallowing, and coughing reflexes) weakened or absent
      - Respiratory failure
      - Clearing the stomach of ingested organic solvents or mineral oil products
   c) Contraindications:
      Acid or alkali poisoning in *advanced* stages with high risk of perforation or evidence that perforation has already occurred; not contraindicated in *early stages*
   d) Technique:
      - Tilted, head-down (15°) supine positioning
      - Decision as to advisability of endotracheal intubation (see p. 255)
      - Selection of a wide-bore gastric tube (finger thickness for adults)
      - Introduction of the lubricated (with water, gel, spray) tube through the mouth
      - Verification of the tube's position by insufflation of air and auscultation of the epigastrium
      - Evacuation of the stomach by drainage and suction; reservation of gastric contents
      - Gastric lavage, recording the amounts of fluid introduced and drained (In adults, each rinsing should be done with 200–300 mL water at body temperature to a total amount of at least 20 L.)
      - After lavage has been completed, clamping off and removal of the gastric tube, followed by introduction of an indwelling nasogastric tube
      - Administration of activated charcoal via the nasogastric tube for adsorption (adults: 30 g)
      - Administration of sorbitol to induce diarrhea

- *Secondary detoxification:*
  To accelerate elimination of poisons once they have been absorbed
  1. Extracorporeal extraction of poisons by:
     - Hemodialysis (see p. 311)
     - Hemoperfusion (see p. 318)
     - Hemofiltration (see p. 315)
     - Plasmapheresis (see p. 324)
     a) Indication is based on:
        - Severe clinical symptoms of poisoning: Progressive circulatory collapse of long duration, deepening coma, and severe, persistent hypothermia
        - EEG intermittently or continuously flat
        - Potentially lethal blood levels
     b) The indication is given if at least 2 of these criteria are fulfilled.
        Demonstration of critical blood levels alone does not establish the indication.
     c) For critical (potentially lethal) blood levels see Table **25,** p. 318.
  2. Hyperventilation in treatment of poisoning by volatile hydrocarbons:
     a) Indication:
        Evidence of chlorinated hydrocarbons in exhaled air with or without typical signs of poisoning
     b) Procedure if spontaneous respiration is sufficient: insufflation of 2–3 L CO_2/min via nasal tube equipped with a snugly-fitted cuff. If $PaCO_2$ is allowed to exceed 50 mm, this therapy must be discontinued.
     c) Procedure in patients undergoing ventilation:
        adjustment of ventilation volume to 25–30 L/min.
        CO_2 is added to the inhaled air (7–10% of total volume) to prevent hypocapnia.
        Therapeutic hyperventilation should be discontinued when there is no more evidence of chlorinated hydrocarbons in the exhaled air, or transaminases fall to 50 mU/mL or less in patients in whom they had been elevated.

3. Forced diuresis makes sense only for substances excreted mainly via the kidneys, and for which there is evidence that enhancement of renal elimination is possible, e.g.:
   - Salicylates
   - Barbital
   - Phenobarbital
   - Lithium salts
   - Thallium
   - Meprobamate
   - Isoniazid

   Remember:

   Forced diuresis is *contraindicated* if poisoning is merely suspected, and in comas of uncertain origin.

- Mechanical ventilation
  Indications:
  - Clinical signs of respiratory impairment (respiratory paralysis; slowed, superficial respirations; accelerated respirations with dyspnea; or cyanosis)
  - Severe poisoning with coma, regardless of blood gas levels
  - Poisoning involving impaired consciousness or unconsciousness and tracheobronchial aspiration, regardless of blood gas levels
  - Poisoning involving threatened or overt ARDS (see p. 109)
- Treatment of shock:
  1. The pathogenesis of shock in poisoning is multifactorial:
     - Volume depletion (due to inadequate intake of fluids, vomiting, or sequestration of fluids in skin and muscle tissue)
     - Impairment of circulatory regulation (inadequate vasoconstriction and relative bradycardia in sleeping-pill overdosage)
     - Diminished cardiac output
  2. Appropriate treatment:
     - Volume replacement with CVP monitoring, in severe cases monitoring of PA pressures
     - Sympathomimetic drugs (dopamine, norepinephrine), if shock treatment with volume replacement alone fails
- Computation of water-electrolyte and acid-base input-output balance to maintain or restore homeostasis
- Normalization of body temperature:
  Rewarming in the event of hypothermia
  Controlled lowering of temperature in hyperthermia
- Prevention of damage to skin, muscle tissue, and joints by physical therapy

- Drug emergencies arise from symptoms of intoxication or withdrawal, or from abnormal psychogenic reaction to drugs. Intoxication results from overdosage.

- Morphine intoxication
  1. Symptoms:
     - Coma
     - Respiratory failure
     - Miosis
     - Pulmonary edema (in heroin intoxication)
  2. Therapy:
     - Intubation and mechanical ventilation
     - Antagonists, e.g. naloxone 0.1–0.4 mg/kg bw IV
     Remember:
     May elicit acute symptoms of withdrawal in drug addicts

- Intoxication with psychedelic agents [e.g., hashish or marijuana, mescaline, LSD (lysergic acid diethylamide)]:
  1. Symptoms:
     - Psychological: acute anxiety psychosis, hallucinations, psychomotor unrest, tremor
     - Somatic: mydriasis, tachycardia, hypertension (in some cases), hyperreflexia
     - Following extremely large overdoses: ataxia, spastic paralysis, pyrimidal tract signs, bradycardia, hypotension, respiratory failure
  2. Therapy:
     - Sedation with diazepam 10–20 mg IV. *Contraindicated:* barbiturates, reserpine, tricyclic antidepressants
     - To counteract tachycardia: verapamil 5 mg IV

- Amphetamine intoxication (e.g., dextroamphetamine, phenmetrazine, methamphetamine)
  1. Symptoms:
     - Psychological: Acute psychosis, hallucinations, mistaken interpretation of surroundings, hyperthermia, emotional excitability, psychomotor restlessness; in severe cases clouded consciousness, seizures, coma
     - Somatic: rise of blood pressure, tachycardia, cardiac arrhythmias, palpitations, headache, outbreaks of perspiration, hyperthermia
     - After extreme overdoses: hypertensive encephalopathy, heart failure, hyperpyrexia
  2. Therapy:
  - Sedation with diazepam 10–20 mg IV. *Contraindicated:* barbiturates, reserpine, tricyclic antidepressants
  - To counteract hypertension: verapamil 5 mg IV

Parenteral Alimentation

Principle

- IV administration of nutrients adequate in calories and types of energy source, amino acid composition, and vitamins *and* adapted to the patient's current metabolic condition, with the goal of preventing or overcoming malnutrition and its sequelae.
- *Total* intravenous alimentation is indicated *only* if even partial enteral nutrition is not feasible.

Indications

- Basically, the indication for IV alimentation is given when natural oral or artificial enteral administration of food is not feasible and/or digestion and absorption are severely impaired.
  The indication depends less on the nature of the underlying disorder than on its severity and complications during the course.
- The indications for IV nutrition fall into 3 categories:
  1. Hypermetabolism with protein breakdown in critically ill patients with acute respiratory failure, acute renal failure, sepsis, coma of varying etiology, trauma, major surgery, severe intoxication
  2. Transportation disorders of the GI tract with or without relief of the GI tract:
     - Risk of aspiration
     - Atony
     - Stenosis
     - Chemical burns of the GI tract
     - GI bleeding
     - Severe, acute pancreatitis
     - Ileus and peritonitis
     - Major surgery
     - Florid enterocolitis
  3. Malnutrition due to:
     - Malabsorption: chronic inflammatory disease of the intestine, severe pancreatic failure, short gut syndrome
     - Anorexia
     - Tumor disorders related to radiation therapy and/or chemotherapy
     - Acute metabolic decompensation: uremia, hepatic failure, severely decompensated diabetes

Constituents

- Carbohydrates:
  - Dextrose in water (D/W) 20–70%
  - Solutions containing dextrose equivalents (fructose) in variable concentrations
- Lipids: Emulsions containing 10–20% soybean oil
- Amino acid solutions:
  1. Conventional standard solutions contain 5–10% L-amino acids. A distinction is made between so-called demand-adapted and utilization-adapted solutions and those based on potato-egg formulations.
  2. Adapted amino acid solutions: amino acid solutions whose composition deviates substantially from standard formulas, and which have been adapted to compensate for specific defects in amino acid metabolism in certain conditions:
     - Trauma solutions adapted to protein metabolism in post-traumatic conditions
     - Renally adapted amino acid solutions in acute renal failure
     - Liver-adapted solutions for treatment of severe hepatic failure

Technique – Dosage

- The infusion protocol for IV nutrition should be drawn up in 3 stages:
  - Establishment of protein requirements, with careful attention to intolerance of specific proteins
  - Determination of caloric requirements and assignment to various food categories, with careful attention to intolerance of certain carbohydrates and fats
  - Determination of water and electrolyte needs

In assessment of protein and caloric requirements, it is useful to assign patients to either of 2 categories:
  - Patients with stress syndromes that demand high-calorie, total IV nutrition: acute, severe illness; injuries or major surgery followed by acute respiratory failure, sepsis, coma, acute renal failure, hyperpyrexia (essentially, category 1 of the indications given on p. 202)
  - Patients requiring full or partial IV nutrition, but for whom hypercatabolism as in the first category need not be assumed (mostly indication categories 2 and 3)

Parenteral Alimentation

- Step 1: Determination of protein needs, with careful consideration of any protein intolerance:
  - Protein requirements in simple IV feeding: 0.8–1.0 g amino acids/kg BW daily
  - Protein requirements in high-calorie total IV alimentation: 1.6–2.0 g amino acids/kg BW daily

Selection of amino acid solutions:
  - As a rule, standardized solutions should be used. Exceptions: protein intolerance, amino acid imbalance
  - In acute renal failure with expanded nitrogen pool and toxic uremic metabolites, mixtures of essential amino acids specially adapted to uremic metabolism should be given. Dosage: when creatinine levels are below 6 mg/dL, dialysis is unnecessary: 0.5 g/kg BW daily; when creatinine levels exceed 6 mg/dL and hemodialysis is required, 0.8–1.2 g/kg BW daily
  - Patients with acute hepatic failure and abnormal plasma amino acid profiles with cerebrotoxic effects of amino acids and their metabolites require specially adapted amino acid mixtures that contain a larger proportion of branched-chain amino acids. The more extreme variants of amino acid mixtures used in hepatic failure include valine solutions and solutions containing only branched-chain amino acids. They are suitable for treatment of hepatic encephalopathy, but are inadequate for total parenteral alimentation.
  - Severely traumatized patients or those who have just undergone major surgery have a so-called post-stress metabolism with abnormal plasma amino acid profiles and protein catabolism requiring stress-adapted amino acid mixtures (i.e., with a low proportion of branched-chain amino acids).
  - Patients with sepsis also have unique amino acid requirements. Appropriate amino acid mixtures are being developed.
- Step 2: Determination of caloric needs and choice of energy sources:
  - Patients on simple IV alimentation: 25–30 kcal/kg BW daily (basal metabolism + 25%)
  - Patients on high-calorie, total IV alimentation: 35–40 kcal/kg BW daily (basal metabolism + 50%)
  - So-called "metabolic computers" for determination of individual daily metabolic turnover are being developed, based on indirect calorimetry in conjunction with mechanical ventilators.

Selection of energy sources:
  - 60–70% of energy requirements should be met by carbohydrates. The basic solution is dextrose in water (D/W). In case of dextrose intolerance, e.g., in post-stress metabolism in critically ill patients or in diabetic patients on IV alimentation, mixtures of dextrose equivalents may be given, or insulin added.

- 40% of energy requirements should be given as fat, with careful attention to lipid intolerances and contraindications for lipid emulsions. Contraindications for infusion of lipid emulsions are controversial. Lipid intolerance by intensive care patients has apparently been overrated in the past. Opinions also differ as to the advisability of administering lipids following trauma or major surgery, or in acute illnesses with post-stress metabolism. Good results of such procedures in acute renal failure have been reported. In severely decompensated diabetes, high-calorie IV alimentation may be feasible only if lipids are included.

● Step 3: Coordination with the infusion protocol to maintain water and electrolyte homeostasis, with replacement of phosphate as required in artificial alimentation (see p. 230).

● In IV alimentation of patients with acute, severe illnesses, surgery, or trauma, caloric and nitrogen needs can be met only if secondary measures to combat hypercatabolism are undertaken: sedation, mechanical ventilation, autonomic blockade, temperature control.

Complications

● Complications related to IV lines; see p. 11.
● Metabolic complications:
1. Carbohydrate metabolism:
  a) Hyperglycemia with hypersomolality and consequent osmotic diuresis owing to glycosuria; risk of dehydration. Surveillance must include frequent monitoring of blood and urinary sugar, osmolality, and diuresis. Prevention by heeding maximum dosages and administration of insulin and/or dextrose equivalents.
  b) Hypoglycemia may develop due to overdosage of insulin or (more frequently) following abrupt reduction of dextrose during transition to lower concentrations as called for by the infusion protocol. Prevention by frequent blood sugar monitoring and controlled, uninterrupted administration of both carbohydrate and insulin with no abrupt changes either of insulin dosage or of carbohydrate dosage.
  c) An acutely life-threatening situation may ensue upon infusion of fructose in a patient with hereditary fructose intolerance. Remember:
  Carbohydrate intolerance is possible for dextrose as well as for fructose.
  Dextrose intolerance in the ICU is most prevalent in patients with post-stress metabolism and in diabetics. Post-stress metabolism involves a peripheral disorder of dextrose utilization with hyperglycemia despite elevated insulin levels. Patients with diabetes mellitus are also at risk for extreme

hyperglycemia, especially undiagnosed Type I diabetics. Life-threatening hyperglycemia may be counteracted by:

- Administration of carbohydrate mixtures containing dextrose equivalents, some of which can be metabolized without insulin, and which have been shown by experience not to predispose to excessive augmentation of blood sugar even in case of dextrose intolerance. Insulin is usually not required in such cases, but blood sugar monitoring is advised as a precaution. If fructose is given, there is a risk of previously unknown fructose intolerance becoming overt.
- Simultaneous administration of large doses of insulin with dextrose. Patients with post-stress metabolism are at high risk for iatrogenic hypoglycemia, since their insulin requirements fluctuate greatly. It must also be kept in mind that insulin has a large range of effects other than lowering blood sugar. Sole use of large amounts of highly concentrated dextrose may also induce hyperosmolar coma.

Fructose intolerance as a hereditary metabolic disorder also develops occasionally in adults. As a rule, the history of adults with this disorder contains a few clues (intolerance of sweets, fruit, and fruit juices; unusually few dental cavities; "sugar allergy"), but may be unobtainable in critically ill patients. Fructose intolerance is much rarer than dextrose intolerance, but it presents a critical problem in that administration of fructose to such patients may be lethal. In each case the ICU physician must make a decision in favor of one of two basic approaches, i.e., dextrose equivalents or dextrose/insulin.

2. Phosphate metabolism:
Phosphate deficiency with hypophosphatemia is particularly likely to occur when high-calorie IV nutrition is initiated abruptly or consists largely of levulose (fructose). Patients with preexistent hypophosphatemia are at risk. For identification and treatment see p. 230.

3. Uric acid metabolism:
Hyperuricemia is a potential threat which may be avoided by monitoring of serum uric acid and adherance to maximum dosages, particularly of dextrose equivalents.

- Organ complications:
  - Cerebrotoxic effects of essential amino acids due to overdosage or inappropriate dosage in patients with acute hepatic failure
  - Hepatocellular damage following abrupt initiation of high-calorie IV alimentation, particularly in case of preexistent malnutrition and large proportion of dextrose equivalents

- Basic rules for prevention of complications in IV nutrition:
  1. Assessment of individual needs regarding calories, protein, carbohydrates, and fats, with careful attention to intolerances and to clues to fructose intolerance in the case history!
  2. Establishment of detailed alimentation and medication protocols
  3. Stepwise buildup of full-range IV alimentation, with avoidance of abrupt changes
  4. Careful adherance to the infusion protocol
  5. Monitoring of the patient's response by laboratory checks at regular intervals, mandatory in every type of IV alimentation
- Recommended maximum carbohydrate allowances per hour:
  - Fructose: 0.25 g/kg BW
  - Dextrose (in post-stress metabolic state): up to 0.300 g/kg BW.

For each dextrose equivalent in total parental alimentation: up to 3.0 g/kg BW daily

Water and Sodium Homeostasis

Principle

- Maintenance of fluid balance in severe disorders (restoration and maintenance of homeostasis) by balanced infusion of aqueous electrolyte solutions
- Prerequisites: monitoring of fluid balance, awareness of typical causes of disorders of fluid homeostasis in ICU patients, and identification of such disorders
- The "water-and-electrolyte" infusion protocol must be coordinated with the "IV nutrition" protocol if the patient is being fed intravenously. Calculated requirements for water, electrolytes, energy (carbohydrates, possibly fats), and protein form the basis for the final infusion plan the physician must order for each patient individually.
- The individualized infusion protocol must contain exact instructions on type of solution to be administered, any supplements, and rate of infusion or time over which infusions are to be given.

Indications

- The goals of infusion therapy are:
  1. Prevention of disorders of water homeostasis and maintenance of volemia by balanced administration of water and sodium as part of balanced infusion therapy (basic requirements or adjusted basic requirements)
  2. Restoration of fluid balance by adding or subtracting computed amounts of water and/or sodium, or by deleting water and/or sodium entirely (= adjusted requirements)
  3. Overcoming dyshydration by treating the underlying condition
- The indications for balanced infusion therapy are therefore:
  1. Deficient intake of fluids, as in:
     - Severe illness or helplessness
     - Unconsciousness or clouded consciousness
     - Severely impaired GI function
     - Anorexia due to illness
     - Artificial alimentation
     - Artificial ventilation
  2. Loss of large amounts of fluid, as in:
     - Severe vomiting
     - Severe diarrhea
     - Persistent high fever

3. Marked regulatory disorders of water and electrolyte homeo-
stasis, e.g., in:
   – Acute or decompensated chronic renal failure
   – Acute hepatic failure
   – Severely decompensated diabetes mellitus
4. Overt, life-threatening disorders of fluid balance

Infusions

- In principle, water and electrolytes may be administered as commercially available electrolyte solutions or by adding concentrated
electrolytes to electrolyte-free vector solutions (e.g., 5% D/W) or
nutrient solutions.

- Classification of the large selection of available electrolyte solutions
with and without carbohydrates is based exclusively on criteria of
fluid and electrolyte homeostasis, regardless of the underlying
condition. The major categories are *electrolyte-isotonic* and *electrolyte-hypotonic* solutions. "Pure", electrolyte-free water is administered as 5% carbohydrate solution. *Balanced solutions* and *replacement solutions* are available for special purposes, as is a large
selection of *carbohydrate solutions containing electrolytes.*

- *Electrolyte-isotonic solutions* contain electrolytes in concentrations
corresponding to normal serum osmolality. They are therefore
plasma-isotonic with regard to their electrolyte content.
1. Isotonic electrolyte solutions are suited primarily for replacement of extracellular fluid.
2. Small amounts may also be used as vector solutions for drugs or
concentrated electrolytes, or to maintain patency of indwelling
venous catheters.
3. Typical vector solutions for drugs or concentrated electrolytes
are normal saline, balanced electrolyte solutions, and Ringer-
lactate solutions.
   – "Physiologic" saline (0.9%) is the most widely used. Strictly
speaking, the sodium concentration is "unphysiologic", but
autoregulatory processes are able to adjust for that.
   – Balanced electrolyte solutions contain sodium, potassium,
calcium, magnesium, and chloride in concentrations similar to
those in extracellular fluid under normal conditions. This is
regarded as an advantage over 0.9% saline.
   – Ringer-lactate solution is similar in composition to the
balanced electrolyte solutions. It is used to replace extracellular fluid lost due to trauma, burns, and major surgery.

- *Electrolyte-hypotonic solutions* contain electrolytes in concentrations below those in normal plasma. Being free of carbohydrates,
they are also hypotonic with regard to plasma osmolality. As a rule,
however, electrolyte-hypotonic solutions are made isotonic to

plasma by addition of carbohydrate. A solution containing electrolytes in concentrations equivalent to half the normal plasma levels is referred to as a "semi-electrolyte" solution. Other special solutions are designated according to the conditions in which they are to be used, e.g., rehydration or "renal starter" solutions.

- "Semi-electrolyte" solutions contain the major serum electrolyte components in half their normal serum concentrations. They are indicated for replacement of extracellular fluid in marked hypertonic dehydration due primarily to water loss.

- "Rehydration solutions" contain NaCl in concentrations below those in normal serum. Most of the wide variety of available rehydration solutions are quite similar to semi-electrolyte solutions. Electrolyte-hypotonic rehydration solutions with a lower electrolyte content (e.g., ⅓-molar electrolyte solutions) are no longer recommended.

- *Electrolyte-free water* can be administered in the form of 5% D/W. Oxidation of the dextrose yields osmotically ineffective "free water". According to the present opinion, electrolyte-free solutions are not indicated for rehydration in hypertonic dehydration. Since hypertonic dehydration usually also involves a deficiency of sodium, simple water deficiency rarely occurs. Moreover, brain tissue is able to adapt to hypertonicity of extracellular fluid by proportionately increasing its own content of osmotically active substances. Shrinkage of brain tissue in response to hyperosmolality of extracellular fluid is probably transitory. Once the brain has become adapted in this fashion, infusion of osmotically "free" water may lead to brain edema.

- *Basic electrolyte solutions* contain daily normal water, sodium, and potassium requirements for an adult in 30–35 mL/kg BW (i.e., 1500 mL/m² surface area). The potassium content is considerably higher than that in balanced electrolyte solutions. Such basic solutions are suitable for supplying water and electrolytes in uncomplicated cases not requiring precise balancing of water and electrolytes.

- *Replacement solutions* for GI fluid losses are compounded to make up for lost volume on a 1:1 basis. The volume of infused fluid corresponds to the volume of fluid lost. Replacement solutions too may be given in uncomplicated cases, or if facilities for monitoring water and electrolyte homeostasis are deficient.

- Solutions designed to replace lost gastric secretions are employed most frequently. They are intended to provide isovolumetric substitution.

- Solutions for replacement of lost small intestinal secretions, which are alkaline, are also available.

Table **14**   Electrolyte stock concentrates

	Cations [per ml]	Anions [per ml]
Sodium chloride	1 mmol Na^+	1 mmol Cl^-
Potassium chloride	1 mmol K^+	1 mmol Cl^-
Sodium bicarbonate	1 mmol Na^+	1 mmol HCO_3^-
Potassium bicarbonate	1 mmol K^+	1 mmol HCO_3^-
Sodium phosphate	1 mmol Na^+	0.6 mmol PO_4^{---}
Potassium phosphate	1 mmol K^+	0.6 mmol PO_4^{---}
Calcium chloride	0.5 mmol Ca^{++}	1 mmol Cl^-
L-lysine hydrochloride	1 mmol $L\text{-lys-}H^+$	1 mmol Cl^-
L-arginine hydrochloride	1 mmol $L\text{-arg-}H^+$	1 mmol Cl^-
Hydrochloric acid	1 mmol H^+	1 mmol Cl^-

- *Carbohydrate solutions with electrolyte supplements,* commercially available in innumerable variations, are largely superfluous. They are intended for balanced infusion therapy and artificial nutrition. In everyday ICU practice, however, it is simpler to supply energy requirements by IV infusion of highly-concentrated carbohydrate solutions plus electrolytes either added as concentrates to the carbohydrates or given as separate drips.
- Electrolyte concentrates in ampoules usually contain the electrolytes in 1-molar solution (1 mL of concentrate = 1 mmol). Added to solutions for infusion, they serve to replace electrolytes and acid and basic equivalents.

Electrolytes of practical importance available in concentrated form are listed in Table **14**.

Technique

Basics:

- The final success of balanced infusion therapy depends on the correct answers to, and appropriate clinical action on, 4 questions:
  1. Is sodium-water homeostasis intact or disturbed?
  2. Does the basic condition lead to impairment of regulation of fluid balance?
  3. Is there loss or threatened loss of substantial amounts of fluid?
  4. In the event of impairment of fluid balance: What type is it?

- The answers to these questions serve to classify the patient's requirements (see Figure **6**).
  1. Basic requirements: water-and-electrolyte homeostasis intact, elimination of water and electrolytes normal; neither case history nor fluid balance suggestive of abnormal losses
  2. Adjusted requirements: balanced homeostasis without abnormal losses, but pathophysiology of underlying condition such that disorders of fluid elimination likely to occur (renal impairment, hepatic failure)
  3. Replacement requirements: homeostasis still balanced, but abnormal, continuing fluid loss either present or to be expected (vomiting, diarrhea, fistulas, drains, perspiration)
  4. Corrective requirements: overt impairment of water and electrolyte homeostasis
- *Basic requirements* are the average maintenance or normal needs. They are based on average normal amounts of water, sodium, and potassium. Administration of basic requirements assures maintenance of homeostasis, provided there are no disorders of regulation

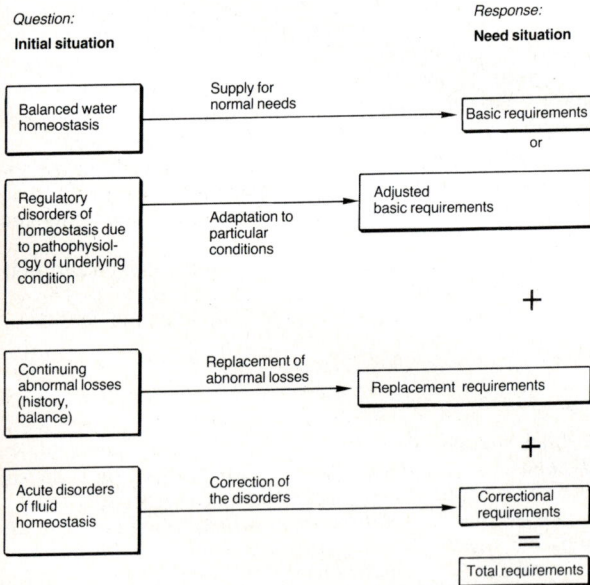

Fig. 6   Summary of input-output balancing of water and electrolyte homeostasis

of fluid homeostasis or fluid content, and no continuing abnormal loss of fluid.

1. Computation of basic requirements:

Water	Sodium	Potassium
30 mL/kg BW/d 1.5 L/m^2/d	80–120 mmol/d	60–80 mmol/d

2. The following are necessary for fulfillment of basic requirements:
   – Balanced solutions (see p. 209), or
   – 5% carbohydrate solutions as vectors, with addition of electrolyte concentrates in appropriate amounts (see p. 210)

- *Adjusted basic requirements* must be met when pathophysiology of the underlying condition involves impaired water and sodium excretion. This is or may be the case:
  – In renal functional impairment and acute renal failure
  – In hepatic failure with or without accompanying impairment or renal function
  – In overt myocardial failure
  – Following major surgery or trauma

1. In chronic renal failure, water and sodium requirements may be enhanced or decreased, depending on the stage. Balancing must be individualized.
2. In patients with acute renal failure, water and sodium requirements depend on the immediate situation, and may vary from one day to the next. Balancing must be individualized.
3. In patients with hepatocellular insufficiency without edema, the infusion protocol should cover basic requirements, but may have to be modified in accordance with monitoring information (see p. 235).
4. In patients with congestive heart failure, sodium and water requirements depend on the degree of compensation (see p. 238).
5. Postoperative and posttraumatic patients have the following basic requirements:
   Water 40 mL/kg BW/d, sodium 250–300 mmol/d, potassium 60 mmol/d. Specially adapted, ready-made solutions have been developed to cover these basic needs in perioperative and peritraumatic situations.

- *Replacement requirements* must be filled in the event of abnormal losses, which can be identified on the basis of the history, current monitoring, and water-and-sodium balancing data:

1. Typical causes of abnormal losses are:
   – Polyuria
   – Loss of gastric juices by vomiting or via gastric tube
   – Diarrhea
   – Drains

- External fistulas or intestinal stomas
- Wound secretions
- Increased insensible water loss in hyperventilation or pro-longed fever
- Repeated attacks of diaphoresis

Abnormal losses of water and electrolytes must be measured or estimated by other means (see p. 217).

2. Replacement needs must be met by:
   - Individualized addition of electrolytes to carrier solutions in accordance with calculated requirements, or:
   - Infusion of replacement solutions, which replenish lost fluid on an isovolumetric basis (volume of lost body fluid = volume of replacement solution)

- *Correctional requirements* are likely when overt disorders of water-electrolyte equilibrium are present and must be compensated by infusion therapy.
- Dehydration is treated by fluid replacement with electrolyte solutions.
- Hyperhydration is treated by restricting administration of water and electrolytes to less than basic requirements and forcing excretion of sodium and water.

Computing the Balancing Protocol

- Setting up the balancing protocol requires recording of intake and losses.

- *Intake* must consider:
  - Enteral administration
  - Parenteral administration
  - Endogenous water production
  - Absorption of vapor from inhaled aerosols

1. Enteral and parenteral intake of water, sodium, and potassium can be assessed precisely.
2. Metabolic water, i.e., the water that is produced by the organism and enters the extracelluar fluid, eludes exact measurement in individual cases, and must be estimated on the basis of empirical data:
   - Water from oxidation (endogenous metabolic water) in adults develops at the rate of 200–300 mL/24 h or 270 mL/m^2, and depends on the energy turnover (10–15 mL/100 kcal = 2.4–3.6 mL/kJ).
   - Oxidation water may increase considerably in hypercatabolic states, but there is no clinically applicable formula for its estimation.
   - If catabolism involves breakdown of body tissues, e.g., muscle, water is formed not only by oxidation (oxidation water),

but also by release of intracellular fluid previously bound in the cytoplasm (preformed water) into the extracellular space.

– In acute renal failure with catabolism, endogenous water production from oxidation and liberated cell water can amount to 700 mL/24 h.

– In severe trauma and infections involving tissue breakdown (catabolic processes), endogenous water production from oxidation and liberation of cell water can amount to up to 1000 mL/24 h.

Remember:

– In critically ill patients with tissue catabolism, constant body weight may be a sign of water retention, i.e., weight loss due to tissue breakdown is compensated by weight gain due to water retention.

– If the weight of a critically ill patient remains constant in day-to-day weighings, one must verify whether this is the desired result of high-calorie, protein-rich artificial nutrition or a sign of undesired water retention.

3. When mechanical ventilators are equipped with atomized aerosols that deliver water droplets to the alveoli, water may be absorbed by the lungs. Pulmonary water uptake of this nature is not subject to measurement under routine clinical conditions. It may amount to 300–500 mL/24 h.

For consideration of fluid uptake by the lungs during prolonged mechanical ventilation, 3 procedures have been suggested in computing fluid balance:

– Entering only half of the assumed amount of perspiration as lost

– Deduction of about 400 mL/24 h (pulmonary loss) from the amount of fluid assumed to be lost by diaphoresis.

– Addition of 300 mL/24 h as alveolar fluid to the measured intake

Remember:

In case of increasingly positive fluid balance or failure to achieve desired negative fluid balance in the absence of evident causes, absorption of fluid from aerosols by the lungs must be drawn into consideration and included in computation of fluid balance.

• *Fluid loss* occurs via:

– Urine
– Insensible perspiration
– Sweat (sensible perspiration)
– Stools
– Secretions drained from the GI tract (gastric and intestinal juices)
– Tracheobronchial secretions
– Exudates or transudates from wounds or in body cavities

1. Renal excretion of water, sodium, and potassium is accessible for precise measurement.

2. Insensible water loss is assumed to be 800–1000 mL/day or 12–15 mL/kg BW/d.
   - Water losses by insensible perspiration are a function of heat loss by the organism; being unavoidable, they are largely uninfluenced by extermal fluid balance.
   - Water losses by insensible perspiration are a function of energy turnover, and amount to 42–44 mL/100 kcal (10.0–10.5 mL/kJ).
   - Fluid losses via the lungs normally amount to about 400 mL/24 h.
   - Use of alveoli-penetrating aerosols in long-term mechanical ventilation alters the pulmonary water balance due to uptake of water (see p. 215).
   - In computing fluid balance, insensible perspiration may be assumed to increase by about 2 mL/kg BW/d for each °C of body temperature above 37 °C.
   - Loss of fluid by diaphoresis (sensible perspiration):
   a) Low-grade intermittent sweating: 300 mL additional loss per day
   b) Moderate intermittent sweating: 600 mL additional loss per day
   c) Heavy intermittent sweating: 1000 mL additional loss per day
   d) Continuous sweating: at least 2000 mL additional loss per day
3. Loss of water and electrolytes via stools may be roughly estimated.
   - Measurement of amounts and assay of electrolytes in stools passed via rectal tube are objectionable from a hygienic standpoint. If stools are merely weighed, their water content must still be estimated. It is usually assumed to be 70–80%, but may vary considerably.
4. Gastrointestinal losses of water and electrolytes occur by vomiting, suction of gastric juices via gastric tube, and intestinal fistulas, stomas and drains.
   - GI fluids lost via tubes, drains, or fistulas can be measured precisely and their electrolyte content analyzed.
   - This procedure, however, involves elaborate care measures, and should be used only in selected, problematic cases.
   - As a rule it is sufficient to measure volume according to the scale on the receptacle, and to assume empirical values in computation of electrolyte content (Table **15**).
5. Aspirated tracheobronchial secretions can be quantified with sufficient accuracy by estimating the amounts in collection receptacles. This is indicated only in patients who produce tracheobronchial secretions in considerable amounts. Assay of electrolytes is unnecessary, and inadvisable for hygienic reasons.

Table **15**   Estimated amounts of electrolytes lost via secretions and excretion

	Na$^+$ mmol/L	K$^+$ mmol/L	Cl$^-$ mmol/L
Gastric juices	60	20	85
Bile	145	5	100
Small intestine	100	5	100
Pancreas	140	5	80
Large intestine (cecostomy)	80	20	50
Stools, well-formed	35	70	70
Diarrhea	80–110	20 or more	50–100
Sweat	60	10	45
Saliva	35	20	35

6. Effusions or transudates drained from wounds or body cavities are accessible to volume measurement. Fistular secretions can be collected in plastic receptacles attached to the abdominal wall. Electrolyte assays are unnecessary; the content can be estimated with sufficient accuracy.

Remember:

The volume of fluid lost via stools and secretions drained from the GI tract, wounds, and body cavities into receptacles can be determined with sufficient accuracy. Analysis of such fluids for electrolytes is rarely necessary; in practice, it is done only when electrolyte balance cannot be restored otherwise.

• Total water and electrolyte intake can be computed by adding the amounts of fluid taken in and subtracting the losses. The balance is the difference between intake and loss.

Remember:

– The most important component of fluid homeostasis is the volume balance. The values obtained are accurate enough for incorporation in the infusion plan.

– Sodium balance: Even when all the above criteria are properly considered, experience has shown that substantial excesses or deficits in the daily balance may occur that cannot be incorporated uncritically in the infusion protocol for the next day. Obviously, this is a critical limitation of clinical balancing.

– Serum sodium levels do not reflect the total sodium content, and therefore provide no information as to sodium requirements. The serum sodium concentration reflects the osmolality of the extracellular fluid. Hypernatremia may accompany a reduction or an increase in total sodium levels (sodium deficiency or excess, respectively). The converse is true of hyponatremia.

217

Serum sodium levels are relevant only when evaluated together with other criteria of fluid homeostasis. If the overall situation involves dehydration and hyponatremia, assumption of a severe sodium deficit is justified. An overall situation involving hyperhydration with hypernatrmia is indicative of marked sodium excess. Hyperhydration plus hyponatremia indicate a so-called dilution syndrome, which is suggestive of severe myocardial failure or decompensated hepatocellular failure.

Infusion Protocol

- The infusion plan for each patient is usually revised at 24-h intervals.
  - The plan must take the patient's current condition (for assessment, see p. 129) and balancing data into consideration.
- In drawing up the infusion plan, 2 situations must be considered separately:
  - De-novo balancing:
    The appropriate amounts for administration to the patient are established for the first time. The balance from the previous day is unknown, and can only be estimated from the history and the attending physician's clinical experience.
  - Day-to-day balancing:
    The balance from the previous day is known, and can be included in computation of appropriate amounts.
- *De-novo balancing:* Prior to drawing up a plan for fluid intake, the following questions must be answered on the basis of current findings and knowledge of the pathophysiology of the basic condition:
  - Is impairment of exretion to be expected?
  - Are continuing abnormal losses to be expected?
  - Is water and electrolyte homeostasis intact or impaired?

Decisions for computation of the amounts for administration depend on the responses to these questions.

1. *First possibility:* Abnormal losses or impairment of excretion are not present and not likely to occur; water-electrolyte homeostasis is intact.
   - Conclusion: assumption that setting maintenance requirements equivalent to total requirements will suffice to maintain balance
2. *Second possibility:* Due to the underlying disorder, altered excretion of electrolytes and water is likely, e.g., in renal impairment, congestive heart failure, hepatocellular failure, or postoperative conditions.
   - Conclusion: assumption of adjusted basic requirements as equivalent to maintenance requirements

3. *Third possibility:* Continuing abnormal losses are likely due to emesis, diarrhea, salivation, elevated temperature and sweating, tracheobronchial secretion, polyuria, drainage tubes, fistulas, transudation, or effusions.
   – Conclusion: assumption of additional replacement requirements, i.e., repletion of abnormal loss by replacing lost components in amounts in excess of basic requirements to reestablish balance (basic requirements + replacement requirements = maintenance requirements).

4. *Fourth possibility:* Regulation of water and electrolyte homeostasis is impaired.
   – Conclusion: assumption of correctional requirements for compensation of the disorder. In deficit conditions, this means administration of increased amounts of deficient components to achieve a positive balance, and in conditions involving excess, restriction and elimination of the overabundant components to achieve a negative balance. In such cases, overall requirements are equivalent to maintenance requirements + correctional requirements.

5. In complicated cases, all partial aspects listed above must be considered in setting up to plan for administration of water and electrolytes: sufficient amounts to cover basic requirements, correct current disorders, and replenish abnormal losses, with adjustments for any impairment of excretion.

- *Day-to-day balance:*
  Continued balancing is based on the balance of the previous day, current clinical findings, and pathophysiology of the underlying condition. The following questions must be answered:
  – Was the balance of the previous day in equilibrium?
  – At the time of computing the balance, is water-electrolyte homeostasis intact or impaired?
  – Are any abnormal losses or impairment of excretion expected to persist the next day?
  Depending on the responses, computation of intake must be adjusted as follows:

1. *First possibility:* The computed balance for the previous day is in equilibrium; there are no clinical signs of impaired water-electrolyte homeostasis.
   – Conclusion: Water and electrolytes are given in unchanged amounts on the assumption that the patient's situation will remain the same on the following day as well, particularly regarding abnormal losses or impairment of excretion.

2. *Second possibility:* Despite correct mathematical balance, there is an uncorrected disorder of water-electrolyte homeostasis.
   – Conclusion: To correct the disorder, administration of water or electrolytes is enhanced or restricted compared to the

previous day, according to the rules for correction of water-electrolyte homeostasis.

3. *Third possibility:* The previous day's balance shows an excess of losses over intake (negative balance).

   a) Loss of water or electrolytes is desirable, as it serves to correct a preexisting disorder (e.g., hyperhydration, sodium excess, potassium excess).

      – Conclusion: To overcome the disorder, a negative balance should be maintained until full correction is achieved. Thereafter, calculation is based on basic requirements or the basic needs modified for continuing abnormal losses.

   b) Losses of electrolytes and water have led to imbalance (e.g., dehydration, sodium deficit, potassium deficit).

      – Conclusion: The disorder must be treated according to the rules for correction of water-electrolyte homeostasis. Furthermore, assuming that the losses of water and electrolytes will continue unchanged the next day, the amounts administered must exceed the amounts given the previous day.

4. *Fourth possibility:* The previous day's balance shows an excess of intake over losses (positive balance).

   a) Retention of water and electrolytes is desirable for correction of a preexisting disorder (e.g., dehydration, sodium or potassium deficiency).

      – Conclusion: To overcome this disorder, a positive balance must be maintained until full correction has been achieved. Thereafter, computation is based on basic requirements or basic requirements modified for continuing abnormal losses.

   b) Retention of water or electrolytes has led to impairment of water-electrolyte homeostasis (hyperhydration, sodium or potassium excess).

      – Conclusion: Treatment follows the rules for correction of water-electrolyte homeostasis.

        Furthermore, assuming that either overadministration or persistent excretory impairment is involved, the amounts given must be less than those of the day before.

Administration of Infusions

- The types of infusions are irrelevant for computation of the water-electrolyte balance. For infusion therapy of ICU patients, for whom individual balancing must be done daily, concentrated electrolytes added to basic solutions usually serve best. It is important that ICU patients be given standardized solutions, e.g., basic, rehydration, or replacement solutions, *only on orders* and with control by balancing.

- Commercial solutions provide the advantage of simple and hygienic handling.
- Addition of electrolytes permits adaptation to individual requirements; the main disadvantage is the risk of contamination.

● Infusions considered in balancing are usually administered to ICU patients as continuous drips via central IV line (see p. 9). Because of the risk of complications incurred by the central IV catheter, the use of peripheral IV catheterization, short plastic indwelling catheters, or winged metal catheters should be considered in patients who are not critically ill.

● The most reliable regulation of the rate of infusion is by automatic infusion pump.
- Automatic infusion always means a pump-equipped system. Gravimetric control systems are just as unreliable as simple roll clamps for regulating the number of drops/min.

Complications and Sources of Error

● The leading complication of infusion therapy in its strictest sense is overinfusion. It results in water retention with the risk of congestive heart failure, in extreme cases with alveolar pulmonary edema of cardiac origin and danger of eliciting or deterioration of acute respiratory failure due to interstitial pulmonary edema, and consecutive risk of brain edema.
- A familiar rule of thumb in intensive therapy is to "keep the patient on the dry side."
  a) The validity of this rule is based on the fact that it is more difficult to get rid of water than to supply it, and that critically ill patients, who have many etiologic potentialities for pulmonary edema, have a tendency to retain fluids in the lungs. Even a slightly positive fluid balance may cause considerable impairment of pulmonary function.
  b) The inherent risk is that hypovolemia may result in circulatory compromise with failure of renal function that may be self-perpetuating. Common treatment errors include administration of catecholamines to stabilize the circulation of patients with a volume deficit, and administration of diuretics or consideration of use of extracorporeal hemodialysis for presumed acute renal failure that is, in fact, due to a volume deficit.

● Complications of infusion therapy in the widest sense of the term include those of the IV catheters: trauma on introduction, thrombosis of the catheterized vein, infection of the catheter, and sepsis.

Water and Sodium Homeostasis

- The most important sources of error in computing the balance and setting up infusion plans are:
  - Overemphasizing laboratory data by neglecting to interpret electrolyte concentrations in serum and urine in the light of historical and clinical findings, pathophysiology of the underlying condition, the previous balance, and intervening treatment.
  - Drawing up a prospective infusion plan based on the balance of a prior time interval assumes constant excretion of water and electrolytes and persistence of any abnormal conditions. If acute changes occur, the balance protocol must be adjusted accordingly.
  - Endogenous water production cannot be computed for individual cases. If too little endogenous water is assumed, too much exogenous water is likely to be given (based on the balance), and retention of fluid may result. Assumption of too much endogenous water results in administration of too little exogenous fluid, with the danger of increasing volume depletion.
  - Insensible water loss may be difficult to quantify. If such losses are assumed to be too high, e.g., in patients on long-term ventilation, too much exogenous fluid may be given, and water retention may occur. If insensible water losses are underestimated, exogenous fluid will be balanced too low, and dehydration may result.
  - Special problems in balancing are posed by sequestration of fluid in inflamed or traumatized tissue, or exit of fluid into body cavities (third spaces). Such fluid is inaccessible for normal functioning of the extracellular space, but this is not reflected by body weight. If sequestration of fluids cannot be prevented or reversed, the amount lost to the intravascular space must be temporarily replaced, i.e., the fluid balance must be arithmetically positive. Fluid mobilized out of the third spaces must be regarded as water of endogenous origin, i.e., a negative balance must be achieved if hypervolemia is to be avoided.

- Even if all available data are carefully considered, balancing is still a rough approximation with many sources of error. It serves mainly to provide the appropriate amounts of water and sodium while avoiding overloads. Fine adjustment of homeostasis is possible only by the body's autoregulatory mechanisms.

Principle

- *Monitoring* of acid-base homeostasis of the extracellular space by analysis of acid-base conditions in arterial blood
- *Reversal* of metabolic impairment of acid-base homeostasis by individually dosed administration of acid or alkaline equivalents *(correctional requirements),* in special cases by elimination of acids or bases
- *Prevention* of metabolic disorders of acid-base equilibrium and *maintenance* of an equilibrated acid-base state by balanced administration of acid or alkaline equivalents within the framework of balanced infusion therapy *(adjusted basic needs).*

Indications

- Metabolic acidosis and metabolic alkalosis:
  - In decompensated metabolic acidosis and alkalosis, the basic indication for correction is given. Each individual case, however, requires a decision as to whether correction by administration of alkaline or acid equivalents is indicated, depending on the nature of the disorder and the overall situation. For example, decompensated diabetic ketoacidosis does not require correction by sodium bicarbonate until arterial pH values drop below 7.20, whereas diabetic lactic acidosis demands correction by sodium bicarbonate as soon as pH values drop below normal. In circulatory collapse the line is drawn at $pH_a = 7.30$.
  - In metabolic acidosis compensated by hyperventilation and alkalosis (arterial pH within the normal range), the decision for or against correction of metabolic deviations (positive or negative base excess over ± 2) must be made for each case individually.
- Continuing abnormal losses of acid or basic equivalents:
  - Abnormal losses of acids are most frequently due to loss of gastric juices. Replacement of acid equivalents at regular intervals is indicated to prevent decompensation of metabolic acidosis.
  - Abnormal anion loss is most frequently due to wasting of alkaline intestinal juices. Replacement of anions at regular intervals is indicated to prevent decompensation of metabolic acidosis.

Medication

- Replacement of alkaline equivalents is usually accomplished by administration of sodium bicarbonate or tris (Tromethamine = Tris-hydroxymethyl aminomethane [THAM]), which act as buffers.
  - Sodium bicarbonate is a universal buffer. It is dispersed throughout the extracellular compartment, which permits good control of its effect by assessment of acid-base status in arterial blood. Undesired side effects may be caused by overcorrection, sodium excess with hypernatremia and serum hyperosmolality, sodium overload in heart failure, and enhancement of CO_2 tension in global respiratory failure (see Complications). Sodium bicarbonate is available in concentrated form (1M) in ampoules ($1\,mL = 1\,mmol$) and as 8.4% solution for use as an IV drip (likewise 1M).
  - Tris (THAM) is dispersed throughout the intracellular space as well. Its intracellular action is regarded as advantageous, but control of the effect presents problems, since pH levels of the intracellular space are not accessible to measurement, and elimination and retention of Tris are also difficult to assess. The risk of respiratory paralysis may be based on an intracellular effect.
  Tris (THAM) is therefore indicated only when sodium must be restricted in metabolic acidosis requiring therapy. This may be the case in:
  a) Sodium excess with hypernatremia
  b) Decompensated heart failure
  c) Hypercapnia in chronic respiratory failure
  Tris is available as a ⅓M solution for infusion ($1\,mL = 0.3\,mmol$).
- Replacement of continuing abnormal losses of anions may be accomplished by adding buffer concentrates to current carbohydrate-electrolyte drip solutions in amounts indicated by the computed balance.
  Lost anions may also be replaced by specially formulated solutions (e.g., intestinal secretion replacement solution). Such replacement solutions are compounded on the basis of volume equivalence, i.e., each volume lost is replaced by an equivalent volume of the solution. Replacement solutions are given when exterior circumstances interfere with exact balancing.
- Replacement of titratable acids is accomplished by giving amino acid hydrochlorides or diluted HCl.
  - The amino acid hydrochlorides used are L-arginine HCl and L-lysine HCl. They are available in 1M concentrated form in ampoules ($1\,mL = 1\,mmol$). To be effective, they must undergo transformation in the liver; H^+ ions are liberated in the process. Efficacy may be impaired by disorders of hepatic circulation or

hepatocellular function. Administration of large amounts to patients with diminished hepatic function presents problems.

– HCl may be infused as 0.1–0.2 N (0.1–0.2 mmol/mL) solution. Carbohydrate or electrolyte solutions may serve as carriers. The H^+ ions thus given act directly, without any prior metabolic intervention. The above concentrations may be given directly as a central venous infusion, but the large amount of vector fluid may have drawbacks in severe alkalosis. Concentrated HCl is available in ampoules (1 mL = 1 mmol).

● Continuing abnormal acid losses may be replaced by adding ampoules of concentrate to the current carbohydrate and electrolyte infusions in amounts appropriate for maintaining balance. Substitution of continuing abnormal losses of acids may also be accomplished with specially formulated replacement solutions compounded on the basis of volume equivalence, so that loss of acid gastric juices is compensated by the same volume of replacement solution. Such solutions are given when external circumstances interfere with exact balancing.

Acid production – and subsequent loss – can be decreased by use of H_2-receptor antagonists.

● Renal elimination of sodium bicarbonate in alkalosis due to endogenous overcorrection can be enhanced by IV administration of acetazolamide.

Technique – Dosage

● Administration is via IV infusion.

● Concentrates (ampoules) are added to vector solutions (carbohydrates, electrolytes, or carbohydrate-electrolyte mixtures). Ready-to-use bicarbonate solutions or those to which HCl has been added may be given via infusion.

● Dosages for correction of metabolic acidosis or alkalosis:

– As a rule, dosage is based on analysis of the acid-base status of arterial blood.

Computation of the appropriate dosage is based on base excess, usually using the formula:

Base excess × 0.3 × kg BW = required amount in mmol (= mL of a 1M solution).

Remember:

The factor 0.3 takes the dispersion volume of the applied substances into consideration, and assumes that the relative extracellular volume is normal. The latter may not be the case; furthermore, the dispersion volume, e.g., of sodium bicarbonate, may vary with the severity of illness. The formula therefore provides no more than rough values. Since the risk of overcorrection heads the list of potential complications, it is inadvisable to insert the factor 0.5 for the dispersion volume.

- Blind buffering is appropriate only in case of cardiocirculatory arrest. The initial dose is 1 mmol sodium bicarbonate / kg BW (maximum dose 100 mmol). If circulatory arrest persists, 0.5 mmol/kg are injected at 10-min intervals thereafter. Blind buffering in the initial phase should be replaced as soon as possible by a dosage based on the acid-base status in arterial blood.

- Dosage in case of abnormal losses:
  - Dosage is adjusted in accordance with analytic data on acid-base status of arterial blood.
  - Dosage may also be based on estimated or measured losses. Control of the dosage by the acid-base status of arterial blood is still necessary, because precise measurement of acids or bases from the content and volume of lost fluids is rarely practicable, and losses must usually be estimated from empirical tables of composition of typical secretions. The same applies to administration of volume-equivalent replacement solutions.

Complications

- Complications of buffer therapy in metabolic acidosis:
  - Overcorrection:
    Overcorrection may result in alkalosis, which carries a risk of cerebral impairment with seizures (due to compromised brain circulation and paradoxical CNS acidosis when sodium bicarbonate is given), ventricular fibrillation, leftward shift of the oxygen affinity curve (i.e., diminished release of oxygen to the tissues).
  - Interference with autoregulatory compensation:
    a) Moderate acidosis causes an increase in cardiac output while suppressing the tendency to ventricular extrasystoles and tachycardia.
    b) The shift of the oxyhemoglobin dissociation curve in acidosis favors release of oxygen to the tissues.
  - Tetany may be elicited in the event of simultaneous hypocalcemia (e.g., in chronic renal failure).
  - Use of sodium bicarbonate carries a risk of sodium overloading and consequent hypernatremia and hyperosmolality.
  - Sodium bicarbonate may cause decompensated congestive heart failure to worsen.
  - There is a risk of hypercapnia if sodium bicarbonate is given in chronic respiratory failure.
  - There is a risk of respiratory compromise and apnea if tris (THAM) buffer is given.

- Complications of replacement of H^+ ions in metabolic alkalosis:
  - Overcorrection
  - Risk of enhancement of amino acid imbalance by administration of aminohydrochlorides in hepatic failure
  - Risk of hemolysis if HCl is given in overly high concentrations
- Prevention of complications:
  - Careful establishment of indications and consideration of the underlying condition and the overall situation. No hasty corrections based on laboratory evidence alone should be made.
  - Disorders that have developed gradually should be adjusted gradually; only those that develop acutely may be corrected rapidly.
  - Blind buffering in adults is justified only in cardiocirculatory arrest; in all other situations, dosage should be based on acid-base status of arterial blood.
  - Uncritical reliance on the dosage computed by the formulas may be dangerous; the effect must be monitored by assessment of the acid-base status of arterial blood.

Potassium Balancing

Principle

- Potassium homeostasis is monitored by regular assessment of serum potassium in relation to blood pH and daily potassium losses.
- Potassium may be wasted by the kidneys or via gastrointestinal secretions. Renal excretion is easily measured, but abnormal enteric losses of potassium (e.g., fistulas, drains, or tubes) can only be reasonably estimated. It is technically possible to assay GI secretions for potassium; however, the procedure is elaborate and unhygienic.
- Potassium overloading results from retention due to renal failure with oliguria. Hyperkalemia is rare if urine output exceeds 1200 mL/day, even when renal function is impaired, provided no further potassium is infused, and potassium-sparing diuretics are discontinued.

Indications

- Hypokalemia or hyperkalemia that cannot be explained by pH deviations alone and fails to respond to adjustment of pH in ICU patients always requires treatment. Otherwise, disorders of cardiac impulse formation and conduction may occur.
- Abnormal losses of potassium must be replaced to avoid the risk of an overt potassium deficiency syndrome.

Medication

- Potassium chloride, potassium acetate, or potassium phosphate are available as 1-M concentrates in ampoules (1 mL = 1 mmol) for replacement of potassium in infusion therapy.
- Dextrose 20% plus insulin will reduce the serum potassium level in hyperkalemia (emergency measure).
- Synthetic sodium- or calcium-loaded cation exchange resins (e.g., sodium polystyrene sulfonate) are available for enteric withdrawal of excessive potassium. The potassium-eliminating effect is further enhanced by concurrent ingestion of 25% sorbitol.

Technique – Dosage

- Potassium may be given to cover basic requirements, to replace current losses, or for correction of a potassium deficit. In infusion therapy, it is administered in the form of potassium-rich solutions or concentrated potassium supplements:
  - Basic potassium requirements: 60–80 mmol/day
    Adjusted basic requirements following surgery: 60 mmol/d
  - Replacement of abnormal potassium loss equivalent to computed potassium balance
  - Potassium administration to offset an overt potassium deficit:
    Total dose: In hypokalemia below 3 mmol/L, 200–400 mmol of potassium are necessary to increase serum levels by 1 mmol/L.
    Dosage per unit time: As a rule, 20–40 mmol/h. More rapid infusion is justified only in the event of cardiocirculatory complications or cardiac arrest due to hypokalemia.
- Potassium elimination:
  - Cationic exchange resins for elimination of potassium: Orally: sodium polystyrene sulfonate or a calcium-potassium ion-exchange resin 15 g plus 50 mL 25% sorbitol q 6–8 h
    Retention enema: sodium polystyrene sulfonate or a calcium-potassium ion-exchange resin 30 g plus 200 mL 25% sorbitol q 6–8 h; effective after 1–2 h, duration of effect 4–6 h
  - Potassium elimination by hemodialysis

The choice of procedure depends on the danger posed by the hyperkalemia, i.e., on serum potassium levels and presence and extent of potassium-induced ECG alterations (see p. 138).

Complications – Sources of Error

- The most important complication of potassium replacement is overloading. Wrong decisions are usually based on:
  - Failure to consider renal functional impairment, especially when potassium-sparing diuretics are given concurrently
  - Failure to consider alkalosis
- Common errors leading to potassium depletion are:
  - Underestimation of basic requirements
  - Underestimation of requirements in patients on high-caloric parenteral nutrition
  - Failure to consider current abnormal losses of potassium
  - Failure to consider potassium shifts due to sequestration of fluid in third spaces, especially in acute abdominal disorders

Phosphate Balancing

Principle

- Monitoring of phosphate homeostasis by determination of serum phosphate levels, assay of inorganic phosphate in the urine, and treatment of overt symptoms of phosphate deficiency
  - Normal levels of inorganic phosphate in *serum* = 2.4–4.8 mg/dL (0.77–1.55 mmol/L). Generally, levels below 2 mg/dL are regarded as hypophosphatemia.

Mild hypophosphatemia:	2.0–1.6 mg/dL
Moderate hypophosphatemia:	1.0–1.5 mg/dL
Severe hypophosphatemia with risk of phosphate depletion syndrome	<1.0 mg/dL

  - Normal concentration of inorganic phosphate in the *urine:* Mean of 74 mg/dL in 24-h collected urine (25 mmol/L)
    Mean daily excretion: 1.12 g/d
  - Phosphate clearance: normal range 10–13 mL/min

Indications

- Replacement of phosphate is indicated whenever serum phosphate levels drop below 2 mg/dL and/or renal phosphate excretion exceeds normal values.
- Phosphate replacement is required routinely in ICU patients with the following conditions, especially if a preexisting phosphate deficit is likely:
  - GI disorders
  - Pancreatitis
  - Hepatic cirrhosis
  - Alcoholism
  - Parenteral hyperalimentation for malnutrition
  - Parenteral nutrition for more than 10 days, especially with large amounts of fructose
  - Sepsis (hypophosphatemia is a leading symptom of this condition)
  - Ketotic acidosis
  - Lactic acidosis
  - Hemodialysis

Remember:
Hypophosphatemia may develop at any time during ICU treatment, but incidence is highest in the initial phase.

Medication

- Inorganic phosphate is available for replacement in electrolyte or electrolyte-free solutions:
  - Potassium phosphate buffer (20-mL ampoule = 20 mmol $H_2PO_4^-$)
  - Sodium phosphate buffer (20-mL ampoule = 20 mmol/mL phosphate)

  The choice depends on the patient's electrolyte status.

Dosage

- Administration is by infusion.
- Concentrate in the ampoules is added to compatible vector solutions.
- The average ICU patient requires normal is 25–40 mmol phosphate in 24 h.
- No more than 0.02 mmol/kg/h phosphate should be given per hour.
- Dosage should be adjusted in accordance with the following laboratory data:
  - Serum phosphate: at least once a week
  - Urinary phosphate: at least once a week
  - Calcium must also be monitored

  Remember:

  Serum phosphate levels undergo diurnal fluctuation, with low morning and high evening levels. Monitoring should therefore always be done at the same time of day.

Complications

- Hyperphosphatemia
- Depending on the type of concentrate given:
  - Hyperkalemia
  - Hypernatremia
- Hypocalcemia

Renal Functional Impairment and Renal Failure

Principle

- If infusion therapy is indicated in patients with chronic renal functional impairment, administration of water and electrolytes must be adjusted according to the severity of renal failure, i.e., the urinary output (adjusted basic requirements).

- Patients with severe acute renal failure necessitating ICU treatment always require balanced infusion therapy and IV nutrition.

- Patients with oliguric renal failure require energy in the form of highly concentrated carbohydrate solutions if overloading with fluids in IV alimentation is to be avoided.

- The acute phase of renal failure is accompanied by a catabolic state and glucose intolerance (post-stress syndrome); this must be remembered when determining caloric requirements and selecting energy sources (see p. 204).

Medication – Solutions

- In polyuria due to chronic impairment of renal function, commercially available electrolyte solutions selected and dosed in accordance with the computed balance are usually suitable.

- In patients with acute renal failure, electrolyte supplements added to current infusions in amounts conforming to the computed balance are best.

- Highly concentrated carbohydrate solutions for intravenous nutrition in oliguria are available as 40–70% dextrose-carbohydrate mixtures (dextrose + fructose + xylitol).

- Amino acid solutions as a source of nitrogen in renal failure are available as specially formulated mixtures.

Technique – Dosage

- Dosage of *water* and *sodium* depends on the patient's condition (dehydration, euhydration, hyperhydration) and the rate of diuresis.
  - For patients with renal functional impairment, basic needs are approximately as follows:
    Fluid requirements   = urinary output + insensible water loss
                             = metabolic water
                             = urinary output + 500 mL.
    Sodium requirements = excreted sodium.
  - For patients with decompensated renal failure and unknown urinary output, the following initial needs may be assumed (provided there are no signs of dehydration):
    Fluid requirements: 15 mL/kg BW/d

Sodium requirements: 0–40 mmol/day (in arterial hypertension 0 mmol)

- In either situation, further dosage is adjusted according to the day-to-day balance, which must be computed at least for fluid volumes.
- In patients with acute renal failure, the daily infusion plan must be set up in accordance with the computed daily balance.
- Overt dehydration or hyperhydration requires appropriate modification of computed fluid needs.
- In patients with *nonoliguric* acute renal failure not requiring dialysis for azotemia, precise balancing usually provides a sufficient basic infusion therapy to maintain homeostasis without risk of water overloading.
- In patients with oliguric renal failure in need of dialysis, hemodialysis should be carried out daily or every other day. If hypercatabolism and/or sepsis is involved, daily dialysis should be attempted. In acute oligoanuric renal failure, hemodialysis is usually a prerequisite for appropriate infusion therapy with IV alimentation.

- *Potassium* is administered in accordance with serum potassium levels interpreted with careful attention to arterial pH.
  - The initial stage of acute renal failure may involve hypokalemia resulting from the underlying condition (e.g., acute pancreatitis, ileus, peritonitis). However, any impairment of potassium excretion mandates caution in replacement therapy, and monitoring must be done at frequent intervals (q 6–8 h in the unstable initial stage).
  - Conversely, hyperkalemia requiring treatment may be elicited by inappropriate infusion therapy or advanced-stage renal failure.

- *Energy requirements* are best met by 40–70% carbohydrate solutions. D/W with added insulin or solutions containing mixed carbohydrates (dextrose + dextrose equivalents) are commercially available.
  - Coverage of caloric needs by fat emulsions in patients with renal failure is controversial.

- *Protein requirements* are met by specially compounded amino acid mixtures (for dosage, see p. 204).

- Use of automatic infusion pumps to regulate the rate of flow is of particular importance in patients with impaired of renal function.

Complications – Sources of Error

- Water overloading in patients with reduced urinary output
- Hyperkalemia in patients with impaired renal function
- Failure to recognize volume depletion as a cause of renal functional impairment (An erroneously low balance will lead to deterioration of renal function due to hypovolemia.)
- Hyperglycemia and hyperosmolality consecutive upon administration of concentrated carbohydrate solutions for parenteral alimentation: avoidable by employment of glucose equivalents and large doses of insulin plus frequent monitoring of blood sugar and serum osmolality
- Enhancement of azotemia due to overloading with nitrogen when amino acid mixtures are given in IV alimentation: avoidable by giving specially compounded amino acid mixtures in appropriate amounts and monitoring serum creatinine and BUN at regular intervals

Impaired Hepatic Function and Hepatocellular Failure

Principle

- In patients with decompensated impairment of hepatic function requiring infusion therapy, administration of water and electrolytes must be modified according to the degree of water retention and any impairment of renal function (adjusted basic needs).
- Patients with acute hepatocellular failure have a tendency to develop hypokalemia.
- Impaired hepatic function leads to intolerance of protein:
  - Impairment of intermediary metabolism alters levels of amino acids in plasma and causes accumulation of toxic intermediary products with toxic effects on the brain.
  - Administration of conventional amino acid solutions may elicit or enhance hepatic encephalopathy.
- In patients with latent or overt hepatic failure requiring parenteral alimentation, proteins are given in the form of specially compounded amino acid mixtures adapted to correct the abnormal plasma amino acid profile at least partially (see p. 204). This permits total IV alimentation.
- Diagnosis of impaired hepatic function is based on clinical and laboratory criteria:
  1. Clinical signs of hepatic encephalopathy:
     - Stage 1 = Impairment of concentration and cognition, slight flapping tremor, hyperreflexia
     - Stage 2 = Delayed response when spoken to; slurred speech
     - Stage 3 = Delayed response to painful stimuli, perseveration, deterioration of speech, clonic seizures
     - Stage 4 = Coma; no reaction to painful stimuli or being spoken to; no spontaneous motility
  2. Laboratory parameters for assessment of hepatic function:
     - Quick's test
     - Plasma activity of Factors II and V
     - Blood ammonia levels
     - Serum lactic acid levels
     - Serum albumin concentration
     - Serum bilirubin levels (poorly correlated to hepatic function)
- Liver-adapted amino acid solutions may be used to treat hepatic coma regardless of parenteral alimentation requirements, although this is a subject of controversy. Special "coma solutions" fail to meet the requirements of long-term IV alimentation.

Impaired Hepatic Function and Hepatocellular Failure

Medication

- For patients with acutely decompensated hepatic failure, electrolytes added to current infusions are best suited to meet calculated requirements.
- For administration of protein in hepatic failure, 5 and 8% liver-adapted amino acid mixtures are commercially available.

Techniques – Dosage

- Dosage of *water* and *sodium* depends on the patient's condition (euhydration, hyperhydration) and urinary output.
  - In patients without retention of fluid, normal requirements may be assumed (see p. 213); if there is a tendency to develop ascites, sodium must be restricted (40–60 mmol Na/d).
  - Patients with decompensated hepatic failure and edema require restriction of fluids to 15–20 mL/kg BW/d and of sodium to 0–40 mmol/d.
    Sodium may be given in unrestricted amounts if no signs of depletion of volume or sodium are present.
  - In patients with severely decompensated hepatocellular failure and dilution syndrome, fluids must be restricted to 10–15 mL/kg BW/d and sodium intake to zero.
  - In all cases, subsequent dosage is calculated on the basis of the day-to-day balance.
  - In some cases of severely decompensated hepatic failure, initial removal of fluid by hemodialysis or hemofiltration may be indicated.
- *Potassium* is given in accordance with serum potassium levels with careful attention to arterial blood pH.
  - Acute hepatic failure may lead to potassium deficiency.
  - Advanced cases complicated by acute renal failure involve a risk of hyperkalemia.
- *Caloric requirements* must be met by glucose infusions. Fructose (or sorbitol) causes depletion of ATP and inorganic phosphate in liver cells, with concomitant inhibition of energy-dependent synthetic processes and augmentation of serum lactic acid levels.
- *Protein administration* depends on individual requirements (0.5–1.5 g amino acids per kg BW daily); individual protein tolerance must be considered when liver-adapted amino acid mixtures are given.

Complications

- Deterioration of hepatic encephalopathy due to infused amino acids
- Failure to identify volume deficiency as a cause of concurrent impairment of renal function
- Inadequate administration of potassium in hepatic failure without oliguric renal failure
- Hypoglycemia due to insufficient administration of dextrose
- Enhancement of metabolic disorders by administration of dextrose equivalents in large amounts

Principle – Indications

- If a patient with congestive heart failure requires IV infusion therapy, administration of water and electrolytes must be adapted to the degree of heart failure (adjusted basic requirements).
- If such a patient requires parenteral alimentation, fluids may be restricted by giving highly concentrated carbohydrate solutions.
- Drips to maintain patency of indwelling IV catheters should run as slowly as possible.
- When penicillin is given IV in large amounts, the sodium content must be considered.
- When albumin infusions are given, low-sodium preparations should be selected.

Technique – Dosage

- Administration of water and sodium depends on the degree of compensation.
  1. For dosage guidelines, see Table **16**.
  2. Patients with compensated heart failure also require careful attention to sodium restriction guidelines in infusion therapy.
  3. In patients with decompensated heart failure, sodium may be infused freely, provided there are no signs of volume depletion or apparent hypernatremia consequent upon volume depletion.
  4. In dilutional hyponatremia (dilution syndrome), which is always a sign of severe heart failure, input of free water must be drastically curtailed. Administration of sodium to correct the hypoosmolality is likely to cause further deterioration.
  In hyperhydration with dilutional hyponatremia (dilution syndrome), the proportion of water in the extracellular fluid is

Table **16** Infusion therapy in overt heart failure

	Na	H_2O
Recompensated heart failure	40–60 mmol	30 mL/kg (2000 mL)
Decompensated heart failure with edema	0–40 mmol	15–20 mL/kg (1000–1500 mL)
Decompensated heart failure with dilutional hyponatremia	0	10–15 mL/kg

excessive in relation to that of sodium (hypotonic hyperhydration), resulting in hyponatremia even if body stores of sodium are enhanced. Dilutional hyponatremia must not be confused with depletion hyponatremia, in which sodium body stores are greatly diminished (hypotonic dehydration). In heart failure, depletion hyponatremia is usually the result of overdosage of diuretics or other forms of sodium loss. Dilutional hyponatremia is always a symptom of severe, advanced heart failure. It develops following acute diminution of cardiac output, usually in patients on a low-sodium diet. Typical causes include:

– Discontinuation or overdose of digitalis
– Infections with fever
– Surgical intervention

In the absence of an acute precipitating factor, the heart failure is in a terminal stage.

Therapy:

– Drastic restriction of water administration
– Correction of potential causes
– Extracorporeal hemodialysis or hemofiltration in appropriate cases

- Dosages based on these guidelines must be reexamined in the light of the daily input-output balance, and adjusted accordingly.

- In some patients with severely decompensated heart failure, initial hemodialysis or hemofiltration may be required for rapid elimination of water. If these procedures are unavailable, water and sodium may also be removed by inducing osmotic diarrhea with 25% sorbitol.

  Sorbitol by mouth: 50 mL q 4–6 h
  Sorbitol rectally: 200 mL q 4–6 h in retention enema.

- Use of infusion pumps to regulate drip rate is particularly important in patients with heart failure.

Complications

- Deterioration of heart failure consequent upon overadministration of sodium

- Diminution of extracellular fluid with signs of volume depletion and depletion hyponatremia due to overrestriction of sodium, usually in combination with saluretic therapy.

- Augmentation of dilutional hyponatremia in severely decompensated heart failure with dilution syndrome due to input of excessive amounts of water

- Increased retention of fluid when sodium is given for dilutional hyponatremia (with the intention of counteracting hyponatremia)

Diabetes Mellitus and Glucose Intolerance

Principle

- In IV infusion therapy of patients with disorders of carbohydrate metabolism, 3 situations must be differentiated:
  - Patients with known, adjusted diabetes mellitus who require infusion therapy (e.g., for surgery, trauma, poisoning, acute abdomen, etc.) = *Infusion therapy in diabetes mellitus*
  - Patients with stress-induced glucose intolerance in post-stress metabolic states requiring infusion therapy with IV nutrition = *Infusion therapy in post-stress metabolic states*
  - Patients reqiring infusion therapy for severely decompensated diabetes mellitus (diabetic coma) = *Infusion therapy of diabetic coma*

Infusion therapy of diabetes mellitus

Technique – Dosage

- Monitoring of blood and urinary sugar levels initially q 6 h, and after stabilization q 12–24 h; administration of insulin in accordance with blood sugar findings
  - In diabetes requiring insulin, half of the previously adjusted amount may be given as a baseline dose to avoid metabolic decompensation, provided the infusion plan provides for an adequate amount of carbohydrate. Alternatively, the required insulin may be given IV or IM only, dosed in accordance with measured blood sugar levels.
  - In the acute phase, when IV infusions are necessary, blood sugar levels of up to 200 mg/dL are tolerable.
- Insulin administration must follow a standard treatment protocol. Various schemes have been proposed; in our experience, the one shown in Table **17** serves well.

Table **17** Standard protocol for insulin administration

Blood Sugar Level	Insulin Dosage*	
	Continuous IV drip	IV bolus
> 200 mg/dL	1– 2 IU/h $\triangleq$ 8 IU/6 h	
> 300 mg/dL	2– 4 IU/h $\triangleq$ 16 IU/6 h	
> 400 mg/dL	4– 8 IU/h = 32 IU/6 h	8–12 IU
> 500 mg/dL	6–10 IU/h = 40 IU/6 h	12–16 IU

* Selected in accordance with blood and urinary sugar levels

- – Insulin administration is accomplished most simply by continuous IV drip. Continuous IV administration of insulin is best regulated by an automatic infusion pump equipped with a plastic syringe.
- Metabolic regulation may present problems in diabetic patients requiring total IV alimentation, assuming caloric needs of about 30 kcal/kg BW/d (as in ICU patients) and administration of sufficient carbohydrate to cover energy requirements (a patient weighing 60 kg would need 450 g carbohydrate). Under such circumstances, up to 40% of energetic needs may be supplied as fat, provided no serious contraindications against fat are present.

Infusion therapy in critically ill patients with stress-induced hyperglycemia:

Technique – Dosage

- Monitoring of blood sugar levels initially q 4 h, and after stabilization q 8–12 h; insulin is given in accordance with blood sugar findings. Surveillance of blood sugar is also mandatory when glucose equivalents are given as infusions, at least initially.
- Insulin dosage follows a standard treatment protocol (see Table **18**).
  - – In the acute phase requiring insulin, blood sugar levels of up to 250 mg/dL are tolerable.
  - – Administration is simplest by continuous IV drip of insulin added to running carbohydrate-electrolyte infusions or via infusion pump.

Infusion therapy of severely decompensated diabetes mellitus (Diabetic coma):

Indications

- There are 2 forms of severely decompensated diabetes mellitus (diabetic coma): diabetic ketoacidosis (hyperglycemic-ketoacidotic coma) and diabetic hyperosmolar syndrome (hyperglycemic-nonketotic − hyperosmolar coma). Features common to both are hyperglycemia and dehydration. The latter is usually hypertonic (serum sodium levels elevated) or isotonic (serum sodium levels normal), although hypotonic dehydration does occur in rare cases (serum sodium levels diminished). In hyperosmolar coma, blood sugar tends to be higher (>600 mg/dL) and serum hyperosmolality more marked (>350 mOsm/L). A potassium deficit may be present in either situation, and assessment of serum potassium is rendered difficult by the influence of acidosis.

Diabetes Mellitus and Glucose Intolerance

Treatment is based on rehydration, administration of insulin, replacement of potassium where appropriate, and administration of sodium bicarbonate in ketotic decompensation.

- Infusion therapy is always indicated in severe metabolic compensation with dehydration, potassium deficiency, GI symptoms, or impaired consciousness.

Technique – Dosage

- *Rehydration:*
  - Initial rehydration with 1000 mL/h of an isotonic electrolyte solution (0.9%NaCl or balanced electrolyte solution)
  - Thereafter, depending on the degree of hydration and osmolality (serum sodium level): 1000 mL 0.9% NaCl or balanced electrolyte solution (serum sodium < 155 mmol/L),
    or
    1000 mL 0.45% NaCl or semi-concentrated electrolyte solution (serum sodium above 155 mmol/L), infused at a rate of 1000 mL in 2–4 h (CVP < 10 cm H_2O: 1000 mL q 2 h, CVP > 10 cm H_2O: 1000 mL q 4 h)
  - Control of CVP and urinary volume q 2 h, serum sodium (and osmolality) at 1-h intervals initially, then q 2–4 h
  Mean total deficit of extracellular fluid in diabetic coma is 8–10 L. Rate of decrement of serum osmolality should be about 4 (2–8) mOsm/L/h.

- *Insulin:*
  1. The low-dose mode of insulin dosage is now generally favored.
  2. Advantages of low-dose therapy:
     - Less abrupt decrement of serum potassium, lower risk of hypokalemia
     - Avoidance of late hypoglycemia
     - Prevention of brain edema consequent upon induction of osmotic imbalance in the CNS.
  3. Dosage in low-dose therapy:
     - Initially, 12–20 IU standard insulin as bolus (optional)
     - Thereafter, 4–8 IU insulin per h as continuous IV drip or intermittent IM injection
     - Blood sugar monitoring at hourly intervals. Ideally, blood sugar should drop by 100 (50–150) mg/dL/h until it reaches 250 mg/dL. At that level, insulin should be stopped, and 5% D/W given by IV drip. Monitoring of blood sugar must be continued, and insulin administration continued in accordance with a standard protocol (see Table **18**, p. 244). Infusion therapy must be continued until the metabolic situation is stable and oral intake of fluids and food is possible, permitting adjustment based on pre- and postprandial blood sugar values in the usual fashion.

- *Potassium replacement:*
  1. Diabetic coma always involves potassium deficiency. With initiation of therapy, serum potassium levels may drop further due to any of several mechanisms:
     - Continued renal wasting of potassium
     - Expansion of the extracellular space due to administration of fluids
     - Entrance of potassium into the cells when acidosis is corrected
     - Increase in cells' uptake of, and capacity for, potassium when insulin is administered
  2. Dosage depends on serum potassium levels:
     - Administration of potassium for hypokalemia should be initiated immediately; if potassium levels are normal it should commence with insulin therapy; and if serum potassium exceeds 5.5 mmol/L, no potassium should be given at all.

     - Dosage:

Serum	$<$ 3	mmol/L	40–60	mmol K^+/h
potassium	3–4	mmol/L	30	mmol K^+/h
	4–5	mmol/L	20	mmol K^+/h
	5–5.5	mmol/L	10	mmol K^+/h
	$>$ 5.5	mmol/L	0	mmol K^+/h

     - Monitoring of serum potassium initially at 1-h intervals, then q 2–4 h

- *Sodium bicarbonate*
  1. Buffering in ketotic diabetic coma has become less popular than formerly, and is done only when the arterial pH drops below 7.2 or 7.1.
     Rationale: Production of ketone bodies ceases immediately when insulin is given, and bicarbonate administration carries certain risks:
     - Abrupt decrement of potassium level with risk of hypokalemia
     - Leftward shift of the oxyhemoglobin dissociation curve
     - Paradoxical CSF acidosis due to diffusion of liberated H_2CO_3 into the cerebrospinal space
  2. Dosage in accordance with pHa:
     - pHa $<$ 7.0   100 mmol $NaHCO_3$/h
       pHa   7.0–7.2   50 mmol $NaHCO_3$/h
       pHa $>$ 7.2   0 mmol $NaHCO_3$/h
     - pH monitoring at 1- to 2-h intervals until normal levels are reached

Diabetes Mellitus and Glucose Intolerance

- For a summary of therapy recommendations, see Table **18**.
- Phosphate replacement:
  Phosphate replacement in infusion therapy of diabetic coma varies widely. Some authors do it as a preventive measure, whereas others are guided by serum phosphate levels: e.g., if serum phosphate is below 1.5 mg/dL, 40–60 mmol Na_3PO_4 are given in 8 h, then continued until serum phosphate reaches normal levels.

Table **18**   Therapy of diabetic coma

Infusions for rehydration	1000 mL 0.9% NaCl/h initially, followed by	
	1000 mL 0.9% NaCl (serum Na below 155 mmol/L)	} every
	1000 mL 0.45% NaCl (serum Na above 155 mmol/L)	} 2–4 h
Insulin dosage	12 U standard insulin IV initially, then 4–8 U standard insulin/h via IV infusion	
Buffering with sodium bicarbonate	pHa below 7.0:	100 mmol/h via IV infusion
	pHa 7.0–7.2:	50 mmol/h via IV Infusion
	pHa above 7.2:	$\varnothing$
	Adjustment of dosage at hourly checks	
Potassium	Serum potassium	> 5.5 mmol/L $\varnothing$
		5–5.5 mmol/L 10 mmol K^+/h
		4–5 mmol/L 20 mmol K^+/h
		3–4 mmol/L 30 mmol K^+/h
		< 3 mmol/L 40–60 mmol K^+/h
	Adjustment of dosage at 2- to 4-hourly checks	

Principle

- Water and electrolytes are administered in accordance with the guidelines for balanced IV infusion therapy.

- Hypophosphatemia occurs in about 50% of septicemia patients; it may possibly be involved in the pathophysiology of sepsis.

- Sepsis leads to hypermetabolism and a catabolic state, along with dextrose intolerance due to impaired peripheral utilization with relative insulin resistance and hyperglycemia. This must be considered when computing caloric requirements and in selection of energy sources (see p. 203).

- In active sepsis, disorders of amino acid metabolism and plasma amino acid profiles have been described as resembling those in patients with acute hepatic failure. The ratio of

$$\frac{\text{Phen} + \text{Meth} + \text{Tyr (Aromatic AA)}}{\text{Tyr} + \text{branched-chain amino acids (Aliphatic AA)}}$$

is markedly elevated.
For this reason, administration of liver-adapted amino acid formulations (see p. 203) has been recommended for fulfillment of the protein requirements of comatose sepsis patients. The interrelationships are not yet fully clear. Specially formulated amino acid mixtures are being developed for IV therapy in sepsis.

- The metabolic disorders persist as long as active septicemia is still present, unlike typical post-stress metabolic states, in which the length of the damage phase (surgery, trauma, infarction, poisoning) is limited.

Medication – Solutions

- In balanced infusion therapy, ready-to-use electrolyte solutions or electrolyte concentrates are given in accordance with computed requirements (see p. 211).

- Caloric requirements are met by carbohydrates to which insulin has been added. Fat emulsions are contraindicated in active sepsis.

- Protein requirements are met by conventional amino acid solutions or – more recently – by liver-adapted or stress-adapted amino acid mixtures.

Technique – Dosage

- Dosage of water and electrolytes is determined in accordance with the input-output balance:
  - Potassium: High-calorie IV alimentation to maintain nitrogen balance must be accompanied by large amounts of potassium (roughly 100 mmol/day).
  - Phosphate: Phosphate 0.5 mmol/kg BW/d should be given regularly; in the event of overt hypophosphatemia, larger amounts are required to normalize serum phosphate levels.
- Energy requirements of 35–40 kcal/kg BW/d should be assumed. The ratio to protein intake should be 140–180 kcal/g nitrogen.
  - If energy needs are met by concentrated dextrose, large doses of insulin may be required to prevent excessive hyperglycemia. The necessary amount of insulin varies from 2 to 20 IU/h, and must be determined by blood sugar monitoring at 4- to 8-h intervals. Blood sugar should be maintained below 250 mg/dL.
- Protein requirements are 1.5–2.0 g/kg BW/d.

Complications – Sources of Error

- Hyperglycemia and hyperosmolality due to D/W infusions; avoidable by use of dextrose equivalents, large amounts of insulin, and regular monitoring of blood sugar and serum osmolality
- Failure to identify volume deficiency as a cause of functional renal failure
- Potentially cerebrotoxic effects of conventional amino acid mixtures given in large amounts in hepatic failure due to sepsis

Principle

- Artificial alimentation via a tube inserted in the GI tract:
  - Stomach tube
  - Small-caliber duodenal or jejunal tube (for tubes, see p. 16)
    GI alimentation is the most natural way of meeting food require-
    ments in ICU patients. Conditions permitting, it should be the
    first-line procedure.

Nutrient Solutions

Presently available diets for tube feeding fall into various categories
with different main indications and areas of application.

- The principal types are:
  1. "Homemade" diets:
     This term refers to nutrient solutions prepared in specialized
     dietary kitchens; they are essentially strained table foods, i.e.,
     natural foods liquefied to pass through a tube. Such preparation
     involves considerable effort and planning, and a balanced com-
     position is not assured. Homemade liquid diets are being
     replaced to an increasing extent by industrial products.
  2. Formula diets:
     Industrially prepared nutrient suspensions are referred to as
     formula diets. Such formula diets are made either to meet all
     food requirements (complete diets) or as supplements for addi-
     tion to normal meals or to parenteral alimentation, e.g., special
     protein mixtures or body-building food components.
     Types of complete formula diet:
     a) Standard diet:
        Standard formula diets are nutrient suspensions capable of
        meeting normal food requirements. They are suitable for
        patients without further metabolic disorders.
     b) Modified or metabolically adapted formula diets:
        For patients with specific metabolic disorders or organ func-
        tional deficiencies, nutrient formulations are available that
        are adapted to the patient's special metabolic needs. For
        example, formulations especially for diabetes or renal disor-
        ders are available. Further metabolically adapted nutrient
        formulations, e.g., for use in hepatic disorders, are being
        developed.

Gastrointestinal Tube Feeding

Indications

- In general, GI alimentation is indicated whenever natural food intake is not feasible, although the clinical disorder and the patient's condition permit GI administration of enough nutrients to cover all the patient's food requirements. In many cases, a combination of parenteral and GI alimentation is appropriate, especially when it is not possible to supply energy-bearing nutrients in sufficient amounts via tube, causing problems of input-output balance.

- Special indications for modified diets without regard to the feasibility of oral food intake are presented by disorders involving malassimilation and/or malnutrition. For appropriate use of specific formula diets according to their composition and the clinical disorder, see Medications.

Medications

- Depending on the constituents and their proportions, there are two major types of full-nutrition formula diets, each with a different indication.

Regardless of the somewhat historical terminology, the two types are:

1. Low molecular weight, full-nutrition formula diets (chemically defined formula diets):
   There is a difference between low molecular weight formula diets of the first and second generations. Low molecular weight diets of the first generation, also known as astronaut, synthetic, or elemental diets, date back to the early stages of industrial preparation of such products, and contain all essential nutrients assembled in the form of their smallest chemical building blocks. This applies especially to amino acids. It turned out, however, that di-, tri-, and oligopeptides are absorbed better than simple amino acids. This prompted development of the so-called second-generation low molecular weight diets, the *oligopeptide diets*.

2. High molecular weight, full-nutrition formula diets (defined-nutrient formula diets):
   High molecular weight, full-nutrition formula diets, also known as defined-nutrient formula diets, are standardized, defined mixtures of natural food derivatives that are industrially assembled.
   The main features distinguishing low and high molecular weight formula diets are summarized in Table **19**, together with differences in digestibility and areas of indication for each type of formula diet.

248

Table **19** Main features of low and high molecular weight formula diets

	Low molecular weight	High molecular weight
Protein	Defined oligopeptides	Milk protein mixture containing casein or soy bean protein as supplements
Carbohydrate	Oligo- and disaccharides	Mixtures of poly-, oligo-, and disaccharides
Fat	Fats containing a high proportion of polyunsaturated fatty acids Essential fatty acids	

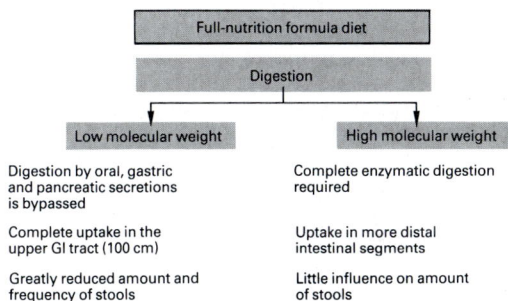

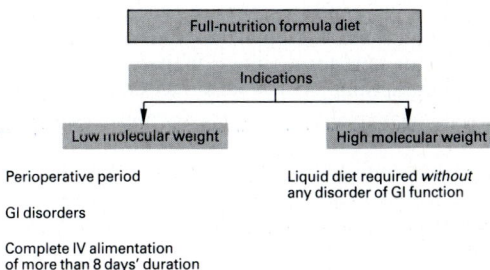

Full-nutrition formula diet		
Digestion		
Low molecular weight		High molecular weight

Low molecular weight	High molecular weight
Digestion by oral, gastric and pancreatic secretions is bypassed	Complete enzymatic digestion required
Complete uptake in the upper GI tract (100 cm)	Uptake in more distal intestinal segments
Greatly reduced amount and frequency of stools	Little influence on amount of stools

Full-nutrition formula diet		
Indications		
Low molecular weight		High molecular weight

Low molecular weight	High molecular weight
Perioperative period	Liquid diet required *without* any disorder of GI function
GI disorders	
Complete IV alimentation of more than 8 days' duration	

Gastrointestinal Tube Feeding

- GI tube feeding is possible via the stomach, duodenum, or jejunum.
  For this purpose, feeding tubes made of pliable, nontoxic material (polyurethane, silicone rubber) are commercially available (see also p. 16). The simplest type of GI alimentation is via indwelling nasogastric tube. In the ICU, however, gastric tubes with too small a bore are unsuitable, since they do not permit suction drainage; overfilling of the stomach with concomitant risk of aspiration is possible in case of intragastric placement.

- Intraduodenal or intrajejunal placement of feeding tubes is becoming more and more the rule in the ICU. For this purpose, a soft, small-caliber feeding tube made of nontoxic plastic is placed via endoscopy. Alternative methods are "active" placement with control by a TV monitor and "passive" placement by natural peristaltic advancement of the tube with intermittent x-ray monitoring.
  In administering nutrient fluids to the small intestine, it is very important to keep in mind that they must be given continuously, since the small intestine lacks reservoir capacity. A nutrition pump to assure continuous flow is suitable for this purpose.
  Remember:
  Liquid nutrients may be given continuously for 2–3 h, then again after a pause of 2–3 h, or continued without interruption. In any case, administration in this fashion is preferable to bolus administration, which has no advantages.
  Catheter jejunostomy:
  Intraoperative placement of a small-caliber tube via catheter jejunostomy. This procedure requires abdominal surgery, and is therefore used mainly in conjunction with operations.
  Percutaneous endoscopic gastrostomy (PEG):
  Endoscopy now permits placement of a transcutaneous tube in the stomach or jejunum without surgery. This procedure is particularly well-suited for long-term enteral alimentation or tube feeding in a private-home setting. Special introduction kits are necessary.

- Industrially processed fluid nutrients must fulfill certain prerequisites:
  - Major basic nutrients present in the following proportions: protein 15–20%, fat 25–30%, carbohydrate 50–60%
  - Nutrient solution containing little or no lactose or gluten
  - Osmolarity below 450 mOsmol/L H_2O
  - pH neutral or slightly acidic
  - Optimum viscosity, i.e., smooth flow and homogeneous distribution

- Avoidance of abdominal strain
- Good long-term tolerance
- Sterile packaging of the nutrient solution

Remember:

Fluid preparations should be given preference, since they are more hygienic and easier to handle.

Complications

- From the tube:
  - Backflow of fluid from a small-intestinal tube into the stomach
  - Regurgitation of acidic stomach contents due to cardiac sphincter incompetence in gastric feeding
  - Aspiration and microaspiration
  - Retention of administered food in stomach when maximum tolerable amounts are exceeded

Remember:

The trunk of a patient undergoing tube feeding must be kept slightly elevated.

- From formula diets:
  - Hyperosmolar and hypernatremic conditions may develop if the nutrient fluid is too concentrated, due to enteric fluid loss.

- The most common complication of tube feeding is diarrhea, which is usually iatrogenic. Important factors that elicit diarrhea are:
  - Selection of an inappropriate formulation
  - Excessively high osmolarity
  - Administration of fluid that is too cold
  - Too much too soon
  - Too-rapid administration
  - Administration of too much nutrient fluid
  - Inappropriate placement of the tube
  - More rarely, bacterial contamination of the nutrient fluid

Note: In case of diarrhea, the possibility that concurrent therapy is involved (e.g., antibiotics) should always be considered.

Remember:

The most important causes of intolerance of tube feeding are selection of an inappropriate formulation and giving too much too soon. For this reason, GI feeding should always be initiated with small amounts given slowly, and the doses increased commensurate with how well they are tolerated. This applies particularly following total parenteral alimentation of more than 8 days' duration, after which low-molecular weight formula diets and gradual increase of the amounts are mandatory.

Gastrointestinal Tube Feeding

- Transition from tube feeding to oral food intake should proceed in a stepwise fashion: Initially, a few sips of water are given to test and train swallowing competence. If the patient tolerates water, he may be given gruel by mouth while the tube is still in place.

Remember:

The risk of aspiration due to gagging is enhanced following intubation.

The gastric tube should not be removed until the patient is definitely able to take food by mouth.

Indications

- The controversy about whether to perform intubation vs. tracheotomy has been clearly resolved in favor of primary intubation.
- Indications:
  - Mechanical ventilation
  - Unconsciousness or neurologic disorders with hazard of airway obstruction and aspiration
  - Retention of secretions and hypersecretion with obstruction and infection of airways that cannot be overcome by other means
- Orotracheal vs. nasotracheal intubation:
  1. In emergency situations, the orotracheal route is preferable.
  2. For prolonged intubation, the nasotracheal route is usually recommended, and is regarded by some authors as the only option. However, nasotracheal intubation is by no means mandatory, and has some serious drawbacks along with its positive features.

     Advantages:
     - Facilitation of oral hygiene procedures
     - Easier fixation of the tube
     - Firm positioning, little likelihood of dislodging or bending

     Disadvantages compared to orotracheal intubation:
     - Technically more difficult
     - Narrower lumen
     - Longer tube
     - More difficult to suction
     - Risk of trauma to the cartilaginous nasal septum
     - Acquisition of bacteria by traversing the nasal airways
     - Risk of bacterial sinusitis

The most important drawback of orotracheal intubation is the loose fit of the tube, which demands particularly conscientious monitoring. Provided good care is assured, we prefer orotracheal intubation for long-term ventilation.

Technique

- *Orotracheal intubation:*
  - Place the patient in a flat, supine position.
  - Flex the patient's head slightly (flat cushion at the nape of the neck) and simultaneously overextend it backward ("sniffing position").

- Insert the laryngoscope with the left hand from the right side, pushing the tongue aside anteriorly and to the left, exposing the epiglottis.
  a) When using a curved laryngoscope, insert the tip of the blade into the epiglottic fold (vallecula), and elevate it anteriorly and craniad. This will erect the epiglottis and expose the orifice of the glottis.
  b) When using a straight-bladed laryngoscope, the blade is inserted so that the epiglottis straddles it, thus exposing the orifice of the glottis.
- Insert the tube with the right hand from the side into the trachea. (The view of the glottis is improved if an assistant uses a finger to extend the corner of the patient's mouth somewhat lateral.)
- Once the tube is in place, inflate the cuff.
- Verify the position of the tube (see p. 255).

- *Nasotracheal intubation:*
  - Position the patient as for orotracheal intubation.
  - Advance the tube along the floor of the nasal cavity to the oropharynx.
  - Introduce the laryngoscope as for orotracheal intubation, exposing the glottic orifice.
  - Advance the tube into the trachea as in orotracheal intubation, using a Magill forceps if necessary.
  - When the tube is in place, inflate the cuff.
  - Verify the position of the tube (see p. 255).

- *Blind orotracheal intubation:*
  - Use this procedure in exceptional situations only, i.e., when visual control of intubation is not feasible.
  - Seat the patient in a semi-erect position.
  - Draw the tongue out with the right hand, while index and middle fingers of the left hand palpate the lateral border of the tongue until they reach the epiglottis, which is then pressed ventrad with the tip of the middle finger.
  - The tube is inserted into the trachea by the right hand with guidance by the left index finger.

- *Blind nasotracheal intubation:*
  - Seat the patient in a semi-erect position.
  - Introduce the tube through the nasal passage, and verify its position by listening for respiratory sounds transmitted to the outer end of the tube: Clearly audible exhalation of air at the outer end of the tube indicates the position of the tube above the glottic fissure.
  - From that position, the tube can be advanced into the trachea at the next inspiration.

Complications

For overview, see Table **20**.

- *Trauma* on introduction of the tube:
avoidable by proper technique, sensitive manipulation, and selection of appropriate tube diameter
Remember:
The tube should be just large enough to glide smoothly through the glottis.

- *Intubation through an inappropriate orifice* (e.g., esophagus, main bronchus):
avoidable by verification of position of the tube by:
  - Direct auscultation at the open end of the tube (in the event of respiratory paralysis, the thorax can be compressed slightly from without while listening for expulsion of air from the tube)
  - Auscultation of respiratory sounds over both lungs
Remember:
Even if the tube is inappropriately located in the proximal segment of a main bronchus, respiratory sounds may be bilaterally similar; but minor movements may cause subsequent slippage of the tube deeper into the bronchus, leading to unilateral ventilation. For this reason, repeated checks of position are mandatory, including:
  - X-ray verification of tube position
  - Marking the exact position of the tube on its outer portion
  - Firm attachment of the tube

Table **20**   Potential hazards of intubation

Complications of inserting the tube
Trauma, bleeding
Inappropriate position
Reflexive disorders:
– Cardiac rhythm disorders
– Laryngeal spasms
– Bronchial spasms

Complications of the in situ tube
Infection
Mechanical obstruction of the tube
Tracheoesophageal fistulas

Complications following extubation
Functional disorders:
– Hoarseness, aphonia
– Disorders of deglutition, aspiration
Laryngeal spasms
Laryngeal edema

    – Positional checks after each suctioning of secretions or change of the patient's position by examination of the markings and auscultation of both lungs during respiration

- *Undesired reflexive responses on introduction of the tube:*
  - Cardiac arrhythmias (in extreme cases, bradycardia or asystole with drop in blood pressure or cardiocirculatory arrest; premedication with atropine usually recommended, although beneficial effect uncertain)
  - Laryngeal spasms
  - Bronchial spasm

- *Complications during intubation:*
  - Obstruction of the tube due to inadequate humidification or insufficient tracheobronchial care
  - Tracheoesophageal fistulas

- *Complications immediately following extubation:*
  - Functional disorders, e.g. hoarseness, aphonia, disturbed deglutition with hazard of aspiration
  - Laryngeal spasms (immediately after withdrawal of the tube)
  - Laryngeal edema (within 24 h after withdrawal of the tube)
  - Vocal cord granulomas
  - Tracheomalacia

- *Tracheal stenosis* as a late sequela after extubation:
  - Serious stenosis affecting function may develop when the lumen is compromised by more than 50%.
  - Damage consequent upon long-term ventilation is now the most frequent cause of tracheal stenosis: Frequency in adults following long-term intubation is 0–3% of those surviving.
  - Typical localization is subglottal stenosis, which is very difficult to treat.
  - Pathogenesis of stenosis:
    The principal cause is pressure trauma by the pneumatic cuff. Infections, arterial hypotension, and high-dose steroids may be conducive.
  - Prevention of pressure damage:
    a) Avoid use of oversized tubes.
    b) Insert a flexible accordion-pleated tube between the tracheal tube and the respirator.
    c) Use tubes with high-residual volume, low-pressure cuffs (cuff pressure <25 mmHg).
    d) Maintain pressure in the cuffs as low as possible = minimum occlusion volume (MOV) = minimum filling volume of the cuff to achieve occlusion.
    The cuff should be inflated only to the extent that sounds of leakage are no longer audible during inspiration. Even if the MOV is only slightly exceeded, a steep pressure increase occurs in the cuff. The MOV must be determined repeatedly,

as it may change with the patient's position and muscular tonicity (i.e., with state of consciousness).

Emergency Measures in the Event of Complications

- *Inappropriate position in a main bronchus:*
  - Slight withdrawal of the tube
  - Intensive endobronchial suction with appropriate positioning and thoracic vibration massage
  - If necessary, bronchoscopic examination (fiberscope)
- *Aspiration:*
  - Tilting of the supine patient with the head down
  - Clearing of the pharynx by suction
  - Thorough clearing of the tracheobronchial tree by alternating suction with thoracic vibratory massage in various drainage positions; checking of the effect by auscultation of the lungs
  - If possible, fiberscope bronchoscopy for visual control of suction
- *Atelectasis:*
  - Careful tracheobronchial cleansing by suction, positional drainage and thoracic vibratory massage alternating with ventilation by a hand-held respirator bag; initial monitoring by auscultation, but x-ray required for verification
  - Bronchoscopic examination with a fiberscope to clear obstructed parts of the bronchial tree by visually controlled suction
- *Obstruction of airways by the tube:*
  - If air exchange is totally impeded, the tube must be changed immediately. If this is not the case:
  - Deflate the cuff and recheck the position.
  - Examine the patency of the tube by suction; if necessary, attempt to clear it by suction. Removal of viscid secretions may be facilitated by rinsing with 0.45–0.9% saline.
  - If necessary, change the tube.
- *Laryngeal spasm following extubation:*
  - Elevation of the patient's head and trunk
  - Atropine 0.5–1 mg IV
  - Administration of oxygen
  - Expectant attitude to observe respirations and general condition
  - If control cannot be achieved by other means, respiration via mask and manual respirator with muscular relaxation; in extreme emergencies: tracheotomy
- *Glottis edema following extubation:*
  - Elevation of head and chest
  - Administration of decongestants (local treatment with aerosols, high-dosed steroids, antiinflammatory agents)
  - Inhalation of aerosols
  - Administration of oxygen

- If still not under control: reintubation; in extreme emergencies: tracheotomy
- *Tracheomalacia:*
  - Symptoms become evident immediately after extubation, as in laryngeal spasms.
  - If respiration is severely impaired, immediate reintubation may be mandatory.
  - Further procedure must be outlined in collaboration with an ENT (ear, nose, and throat) specialist.

Remember:

Differentiation of laryngeal spasms, laryngeal edema, and tracheomalacia can be accomplished by laryngoscopy.

Indications

- The dispute concerning tracheotomy vs. intubation has been clearly resolved in favor of primary intubation.
- Indications for tracheotomy are:
  1. Intubation technically not feasible (primary tracheotomy):
     - Acid burns
     - Massive laryngeal edema
     - Laryngeal trauma
     - Severe facial injuries
  2. Mechanical ventilation of fully conscious patients for very extended periods:
     Secondary tracheotomy after initial intubation may be considered if mechanical ventilation is to last for several weeks. (Conscious patients tolerate a tracheostomy considerably better.) This is most often the case in:
     - Neuromuscular respiratory paralysis (polyneuroradiculitis, myasthenia gravis)
     - Acute exacerbation of chronic airway obstruction with cor pulmonale
- Otherwise, intubation is the first-choice procedure even for long-term mechanical ventilation, thanks to modern tracheal tubes. Secondary tracheotomy is required only in exceptional cases, e.g., when maintenance of tracheobronchial hygiene via the tube is otherwise too difficult.
  - This is particularly likely in severe ARDS, severe pneumonia, and thoracic trauma.
  - In our own patients on long-term ventilation the tracheotomy rate has decreased from 80% to 5%.
- Complications and late sequelae occur less frequently following long-term intubation than after tracheotomy.

Complications

- Large compilations of published statistics indicate a mean complication rate of 24% of tracheotomied patients (10–60%), with lethal complications in 1 8% (0.5–5%), and a mean rate of potentially lethal erosive bleeding of 1% (0.5–2%). Tracheoesophageal fistulas were reported in 0.5–2%.
- An overview of complications is presented in Table **21**.
- Complications observed in medical ICU patients are summarized in Table **22**.

Table **21**   Complications of tracheotomy as compiled from published data

Type of complication	Mean incidence (%)
Infections Local inflammation of tracheostomy Severe hemorrhagic or purulent tracheobronchitis Bronchopneumonia (12%) Mediastinitis	22
Pneumothorax	
Subcutaneous emphysema	
Mediastinal emphysema	
Hemorrhage Intra- and postoperative hemorrhage Postoperative bleeding from tracheostomy (2.4%) Erosive bleeding (1.1%)	4
Mechanical obstruction of the cannula Obstruction by secretions or blood Obstruction by pneumatic cuff Stenosis due to prolapse of the tracheal wall	4.8
Tracheoesophageal fistulas	1.2
Tracheal stenosis Scarring Granulomas Tracheomalacia	5–20

- Conducive factors and prevention:
  - Emergency tracheotomy: Because of the high rate of complications, this procedure should be avoided.
  - Site of tracheotomy: A typical complication of superior tracheotomy is stenosis from trauma to the cricoid (annular cartilage); the most important complications of inferior tracheotomy are erosive bleeding and mediastinitis.
  - Type of cannula: Silver cannulas are well tolerated by tissues and have a small external diameter, but they often cause pressure damage due to their nonanatomic, circular-arc shape. Anatomically shaped flexible cannulas made of wire-supported plastic and equipped with a pneumatic cuff evoke fewer complications.

Table **22** Complications of tracheotomy in patients in a medical ICU

Type of complication	Incidence (%)
Tracheotomy operation	
Immediately postoperative bleeding from the tracheostomy	2
Tracheostomy	
Postoperative hemorrhage	10
Localized wound infection	8
Localized necrosis with dilation of the tracheostomy and/or tracheomalacia	24
Pneumothorax	4
Subcutaneous emphysema	2
Tracheal cannula	
Obstruction of cannula by the cuff	2
Defective pneumatic cuff	14
Tracheobronchial tree	
Hemorrhagic or purulent tracheitis or tracheobronchitis	64
Circumscribed pressure ulceration	8
Bronchopneumonia	42
Major blood vessels	
Erosive bleeding	2

- Tracheal stenosis as a late sequela:
  1. Incidence: In 5–20% of survivors the tracheal lumen is compromised by more than 50% (data from published reports).
  2. The most important mechanisms are pressure trauma by the pneumatic cuff and the cannula itself. Infections, arterial hypotension, and high-dosed steroids are conducive.
  3. Prevention:
     - Avoidance of cannulas that are too large in diameter
     - Use of highly flexible cannulas
     - Interposition of a flexible, accordion-pleated tube between the cannula and the ventilation apparatus
     - Minimum occlusive pressure in the pneumatic cuff (see p. 256)

Immediate Measures in the Event of Complications

- Aspiration (see p. 257)
- Atelectasis (see p. 257)
- Occlusion of airways (see p. 257)
- Erosive bleeding:
  - Removal of the cannula
  - Compression of the bleeding site with the index finger inserted through the tracheostoma
  - Immediate intubation by a second person
  - As the tube is inserted, gradual withdrawal of the finger and inflation of the pneumatic cuff at the level of the bleeding site to compress it; if venous bleeding persists, continuation of digital compression
  - Thorough clearance of the tracheobronchial tree by suction
  - Replacement of lost blood
  - Thoracotomy with exposure and surgical repair of the eroded site

Nursing Aspects

- Care of the tracheostoma:
  - Following tracheotomy, the dressing and the cannula should be left undisturbed for 48 h. Any changes of the cannula within that time should be performed only by the attending surgeon.
  - Thereafter, the tracheostomy should be cleansed daily and a sterile dressing applied.
  - If a silver cannula is used, the inner cannula should be cleansed.
  - If a plastic cannula without an inner cannula is used, it must be changed daily, commencing 3–5 days after the operation.
  - The following factors should be examined in daily care of the tracheostomy:
    a) proper position of the cannula;
    b) patency of the cannula;
    c) intactness of the pneumatic cuff;
    d) inflammation of the tracheostoma;
    e) bleeding from the wound;
    f) subcutaneous emphysema.
- Hemorrhage:
  Postoperative bleeding should not occur later than 6 h after tracheotomy, provided coagulation is normal. Procedures in the event of severe postoperative bleeding from the wound:
  - Compression of the wound by the surgeon
  - Assessment of coagulation and correction of any disorders
  - If bleeding is profuse: careful inflation of the cuff, followed by endotracheal suction to prevent aspiration

- Subcutaneous emphysema
  Procedures in the event of massive subcutaneous emphysema:
  - Open the cutaneous sutures of the tracheotomy wound on both sides of the cannula, and spread the wound edges with forceps.
  - If subcutaneous emphysema spreads to the superior thoracic aperture and the face, relief may be provided by insertion of large-bore needles.

- Tracheobronchial suction:
  - Use sterile, disposable catheters made of soft plastic and equipped with a smooth tip.
  - During application of suction, the catheter should be withdrawn slowly and constantly with spiralling motion; back-and-forth movements should be avoided.
  - Adjust strength of suction manually via a Y-shaped insert; suction should not exceed 40 cm H_2O. Highly viscid mucous may be loosened by instilling 10 ml diluted saline prior to applying suction.
  - Clearance efficacy should be checked by auscultation.
  - To avoid hypoxia during suction in patients undergoing mechanical ventilation:
    a) limit duration of suction procedure to 30 s;
    b) have patient hyperventilate with pure O_2 for 1 min prior to suction;
    c) compensate for lost air by increasing the ventilation volume during the suction procedure.

Mechanical Ventilation

Principle

- Machine-controlled artificial respiration via endotracheal or tracheal tube is used in the treatment of any of several pulmonary and extrapulmonary disorders involving respiratory complications.
- Sophisticated equipment permits modes of ventilation that deviate intentionally from normal spontaneous respiration. The purpose of such modes of ventilation is adaptation to the specific needs of the individual patient and his particular complications by appropriate selection of apparatus and ventilation pattern, to avoid prolonging mechanical ventilation, and to provide for a gentle transition to spontaneous breathing (i.e., weaning).
- Initiation and termination of mechanical ventilation must not be dictated exclusively by blood gas levels and mechanics of respiration, but rather must also be regarded in the light of the patient's overall situation.

Indications

- Indications for mechanical ventilation and choice of type of ventilation must consider the following factors:
  - The patient's underlying disorder
  - Potential and actual complications
  - Extent of respiratory impairment (as revealed by blood gas analysis)
  - Signs of impaired respiratory function, or increased work and frequency of respiration
  - Extent of mechanical respiratory impairment, as revealed by compliance, functional residual capacity, and vital capacity
  - Clinical findings, including chest x-rays
- The indications for mechanical ventilation are not cut-and-dry; they must be determined individually on the basis of frequent monitoring.
- The following summary is intended as an aid to orientation in establishing indications; it assumes that prompt initiation of mechanical ventilation can help prevent further intra- and extrapulmonary complications.

Indications for mechanical ventilation

I. *Absolute indications for mechanical ventilation* (*First-rank* indications)
1. Cardiocirculatory arrest following cardiopulmonary resuscitation
2. Stage III or IV coma
3. Poisoning by organic phosphates

4. Peripheral or central neurogenic respiratory paralysis
5. Intoxication by respiratory poisons
6. $PaO_2 < 45$ mmHg despite 6 L O_2/min via oxygen prongs, regardless of age
7. $PaCO_2 > 80$ mmHg, regardless of patient's age
8. Therapy-resistant tachypnea > 35/min

II. *Potential indications dependent on the underlying disorder (Second-rank* indications: disorder-related indications)
1. Acute exogenous poisoning
2. Polytrauma
3. Major surgery
4. Burns
5. Severe primary pneumonias, including viral pneumonia
6. Drowning
7. Acute hemorrhagic-necrotic pancreatitis
8. Pulmonary artery embolism
9. Immune disorders with pulmonary involvement

III. *Potential indications related to the patient's condition (Third-rank* indications: complication-related indications)
1. Aspiration
2. Septicemia of any origin
3. Circulatory shock of any origin
4. Complicated, acute renal failure
5. Severe metabolic acidosis or alkalosis that fails to respond to therapy within 6 h (pH < 7 or > 7.8)
6. Hyperlactacidemia and lactic acidosis (lactic acid > 4 mmol/L)
7. Disorders of breathing mechanics, including pleural effusions
8. PaO_2 below normal for the patient's age while breathing ambient air
9. $PaCO_2 > 50$ mmHg
10. Diminished total thoracic complicance (< 40 mL/cm H_2O)

- Mechanical ventilation is indicated in the presence of a single first-rank indication (category I) or at least 2 potential second- or third-rank indications (categories II and III, resp.).

- If possible, i.e., if the patient is conscious when ventilation is initiated, he should be informed, then given sedatives. Sedation and endotracheal intubation constitute significant intervention, and require optimum prior stabilization of cardiocirculatory events.

- Contrary to former views, it is now generally accepted that patients undergoing mechanical ventilation should be permitted to breathe actively as much as possible.

Mechanical Ventilation

Equipment

- Two types of ventilator are available; they function according to different principles:
1. Pressure-controlled ventilators with adjustable flow: Ambient air or an air-O_2 mixture is delivered to the patient at a controllable flow speed until pressure drops to a preset level. At that point a valve opens to permit passive expiration.

  Both assisted and controlled ventilation are possible with such machines.

  They are also equipped with a nebulizer system.

  The following appraisal is based on objective experience:
  - Easily adaptable to the patient's own breathing rhythm
  - Suitable for nebulizer therapy
  - Suitable for short-term ventilation in the event of central respiratory depression without pulmonary insufficiency or involvement of extrapulmonary organs (e.g., in case of moderate intoxication for short-term ventilation in patients with bronchial obstruction and moderate intoxication)
  - Suitable for noncomatose patients with neurogenic ventilation impairment in the absence of multiple organic function disorders
  - Highly useful during weaning from ventilation
2. Electronically or microprocessor-controlled, volume-regulated ventilators:

  Such ventilators are designed for controlled and assisted ventilation.

  Various ventilation- and spontaneous respiration patterns are possible.

  The most appropriate type and pattern of ventilation depends on the patient's disorder. Most desirable is active participation by the patient, eliminating the exhausting work of breathing, while maintaining an optimal ratio of ventilation to diffusion.

  This is possible only by consistent monitoring and corresponding modification of the ventilation pattern. Stringent rules are therefore useless, especially since modern ventilators have widely differing capabilities.

  The following is a presentation of the types of ventilation and the terminology.

Machine-oriented ventilation (mandatory ventilation):

Adjustable tidal volume is defined according to time.

a) Without synchronization to the patient:

IPPV	=	Intermittent positive-pressure ventilation
CPPV	=	Continuous positive-pressure ventilation
PNPV	=	Positive-negative pressure ventilation

b) Synchronized to the patient's breathing:

IPPB	=	Intermittent positive-pressure breathing
CPPB	=	Continuous positive-pressure breathing
SIPPV	=	Synchronized intermittent positive-pressure ventilation
SCPPV	=	Synchronized continuous positive-pressure ventilation

Patient-oriented ventilation (spontaneous ventilation):

Respiration times and volumes of respired gases are determined by the patient.

a) ZAP = Zero airway pressure
   CPAP = Continuous positive airway pressure
   (The patient breathes spontaneously and must perform the required ventilation work himself.)

b) ASV = Assisted spontaneous ventilation
   or
   ASB = Assisted spontaneous breathing
   (The patient is provided with "breathing assistance", in order to make spontaneous respiration more effective and deeper.)

Combinations of mandatory and spontaneous ventilation are:

   IMV = Intermittent mandatory ventilation
   or
   SIMV = Synchronized intermittent mandatory ventilation
   or
   MMV = Mandatory minute ventilation
   or
   SMMV = Synchronized mandatory minute ventilation.

All these modes require spontaneous respiratory activity on the part of the patient.

In *IMV* the number of breaths, and thus the interval between mechanical pushes, is defined by the frequency setting. At the end of each breath cycle, the patient can demand additional air as needed. *SIMV* refers to synchronization of the action of the ventilating apparatus to the patient's inspiration.

In *MMV*, respiration is assisted only if the patient's minute volume decreases to a preset minimum.

Mechanical Ventilation

Medication

- Sedation and analgesia:
  Patients undergoing mechanical ventilation usually require sedation and/or analgesia, unless they are unconscious.
  - Patients undergoing patient-oriented (assisted) ventilation may require only small amounts of sedatives and/or analgesics, given as needed rather than at regular intervals (e.g., diazepam, midazolam or fentanyl).
  - Patients undergoing machine-oriented (mandatory) ventilation should be given enough sedatives/analgesics to permit toleration of the ventilation pattern and other care manipulations, while still enabling communication when the patient is spoken to or directly touched.

  In the ICU, sedatives and analgesics must fulfill certain requirements:
  - Rapid onset of efficacy and good control
  - Minimum hemodynamic effects
  - Brief half-life and no accumulation
  - Low potential for addiction
  - Retrograde amnesia

  These prerequisites are fulfilled by sedation with benzodiazepines with short half-lives, e.g., midazolam. Dosage must be individualized, possibly in a definite rhythm. Analgesics may be given in alternation with sedatives, e.g., fentanyl.
  - A combination of fentanyl and midazolam may also be given by perfusion pump:
    Combine 1.5 mg fentanyl = 30 mL and 90 mg midazolam = 18 mL in a perfusion pump. Individualized dosage is achieved with a pump setting of 2 mL/h to a maximum of 8 mL/h.

- Muscular relaxants can and should be avoided to the greatest possible extent.
  If relaxation cannot be avoided (in our experience, particularly following abdominal or thoracic surgery complicated by infection or sepsis), pancuronium 0.1–1 mg at 30-min intervals (brief half-life), following an initial bolus and basic sedation, is appropriate.
  Pancuronium may also be injected into a central venous catheter without ill effects.

- Humidification of the air and nebulization of medication:
  1. Normal air humidity must be supplied artificially in patients undergoing ventilation. Different possibilities are:
     - Spray nebulizers. These produce homogeneous aerosols capable of penetrating to deep airways, but only when suitable apparatus is used.
     - Ultrasonic nebulizers. These are more effective than spray nebulizers, but atomize considerable volumes of water in the process.

- Steam atomizers. These are useful, provided the inhaled air still has a temperature of 37°C at the opening of the ventilation tube.
2. All atomizers or nebulizers are potential sources of infection. Strict hygienic precautions and exchange of tubal and atomizer systems q 12 h are mandatory.
3. Medicated aerosols are reserved for specific indications:
   - Bronchial dilators and bronchosecretolytic agents are indicated for bronchial obstruction.
   - Corticosteroid aerosols have restricted indications (allergic airway diseases, acute bronchial obstruction), and are more difficult to control than systemic treatment, which is also effective.

     Application of antibiotics as aerosols is inappropriate, and is useful only in combination with systemic antibiotics in therapy of bronchiectasis, if at all.

     Application of aerosolized fungicides is controversial; in *mycotic infections* it certainly provides no alternative to systemic administration of fungicides. The mere presence of fungi in the tracheobronchial tree without signs of inflammation is not an indication for fungicides.

Technique

- Regulation of respiratory mechanics starts with a basic setting, which is adjusted in accordance with blood gas findings and hemodynamic parameters.
1. Basic setting:
   - Minute volume (MV) = about 150 mL/min/kg BW (e.g., for a 70-kg patient about 10 L/min).

     This value is computed from approximate CO_2 production (in a stressful situation about 3.5 mL/kg BW/min) and a CO_2 concentration in exhaled air of about 2–3% ($PaCO_2$ = 40 mmHg), using the formula:

$$MV = \frac{3.5 \text{ mL/kg BW/min}}{2.5 \text{ mL/100 mL}} - 140 \text{ mL/min/kg BW}$$

   - Respiration rate: Distribution of minute volume over 8–10 respirations/min (about 15 mL/kg BW *tidal* volume) is a useful base. On this assumption:

     Respiration rate = 8–10/min
     Tidal volume   =   15 mL/kg BW
     Minute volume   =   150 mL/min/kg BW

2. The appropriate values must first be set, then checked by spirometry.

Mechanical Ventilation

- Regardless of the above, the O_2 concentration of inhaled air should be set between that of ambient air and 100%.

  In volume-controlled ventilation, particularly for ARDS or disorders predisposing to ARDS, ventilation should commence with 100% O_2 for 15–30 min to assess respiratory function (determination of I-aDO_2 with F_{IO2} 1.0), followed by stepwise reduction.

  Concurrently, sufficient oxygenation should be strived for by altering the mechanics of ventilation. For example:
  - Increasing the tidal volume
  - Varying the respiratory rate
  - Combination of the above
  - Inflation hold
  - PEEP ventilation

  1. Early initiation of PEEP ventilation is indicated in all types of respiratory impairment involving multiple organ complications, all types of ARDS, and all disorders potentially conducive to ARDS.
  2. PEEP acts to:
     - inflate the alveoli and increase the functional residual capacity (FRC);
     - reduce pulmonary vascular resistance (PVR);
     - increase compliance (C).
  3. If initiated early, a PEEP of 4–10 cm H_2O is usually sufficient.

     The selection of optimum PEEP serves to achieve optimum pulmonary gas exchange.

     Clinically relevant hemodynamic effects (reduction of cardiac output or blood pressure) are corrected by volume replacement or infusion of dopamine (200–400 µg/min).

     Diminished urine output due to renal blood distribution can be corrected by furosemide 80–120 mg/24 h, in divided doses q 4–6 h, if not already overcome by dopamine.

  Remember:

  PEEP is feasible and desirable in both patient-oriented (spontaneous) and machine-oriented (mandatory) mechanical ventilation.

Complications

- Hypoventilation due to leakage or disconnection of the tubing-nebulizer-ventilator system
- Atelectasis due to bronchial obstruction, or microatelectasis
- Infections
- Pressure trauma to the lungs with pneumothorax due to excessive pressure in the airways (An acutely dangerous complication is tension pneumothorax during high-pressure ventilation.)

- Potential toxicity of O_2 in high concentrations, dependent on the duration of exposure; relevant when $F_{IO2} > 0.6$ is given for several days
- Respiratory deterioration in asymmetrical pulmonary disorders due to abnormal distribution of inhaled air (overinflation of healthy portions) or perfusion (hyperperfusion of diseased portions)

Weaning From Ventilation

- The weaning phase comprises the entire withdrawal period from full ventilation to removal of the tube.
- Weaning must be done individually, and depends greatly on the duration and type of prior ventilation and the underlying disorder.
  The transition to completely spontaneous respiration must be *gradual* to assure circulatory adaptation and to provide the patient with a chance to practice breathing.
- The following methods of weaning are feasible and practical after titrated reduction of sedation/analgesia:
  1. *Intermittent disconnection:*
     3–5 min at first, with stepwise increase depending on pulmonary and extrapulmonary criteria. Tolerance is better following transition from a volume-controlled to a pressure-flow-controlled apparatus.
  2. Intermittent disconnection with ventilation under CPAP.
  3. IMV or MMV with or without support of the patient's own respiration.
- Initiation of weaning has certain pulmonary and extrapulmonary prerequisites:
  1. Pulmonary criteria for initiation of weaning:
     - $PaO_2 > 60$ mmHg while breathing ambient air
     - Adequate oxygenation at $F_{IO2} = 0.3$ to 0.4 (maximum)
     - Vital capacity over 20 mL/kg
     - $V_D/V_T < 0.6$
     - End-inspiratory pressure (EIP) < 30 cm H_2O
     - Total thoracic compliance > 40 mL/cm H_2O
     - Unhindered, adequate respiratory excursions
     - No evidence of fresh or widespread alveolar or interstitial pulmonary infiltrations on chest x-ray
  2. Extrapulmonary criteria for initiation of weaning:
     - Stable overall clinical condition
     - Balanced metabolic situation
     - Adequate control of the underlying disorder and complications thereof (e.g., renal failure, severe infections, healing after major surgery)

- Weaning from a ventilator requires careful supervision and flexibility. It should not coincide with other major therapeutic procedures, e.g., intestinal stimulation or hemodialysis as weaning is begun.
- Once the above criteria are fulfilled, weaning may proceed in increments while monitoring the following:
  - Level of consciousness and responsiveness
  - Blood pressure, heart rate, cardiac rhythm
  - Respiration rate and minute volume

  Weaning must be interrupted immediately if the patient's condition is characterized by:
  - Physical exhaustion due to respiratory work
  - Respiratory rate >35/min for long periods
  - Lack of sufficient tidal volume
  - Hypotension, disorders of heart rate, or cardiac arrhythmias
  - Clouding of consciousness
  - Increasing arterial hypoxemia during spontaneous respiration despite administration of O_2
  - Deterioration of the overall clinical picture or metabolic situation in the further course of weaning (e.g., fever or hyperlactacidemia)
- Extubation may proceed when:
  - the patient has been breathing ambient air or a maximum or 3 L O_2/min spontaneously for several hours without complications;
  - the patient's overall pulmonary and extrapulmonary situation is stable;
  - the patient is sufficiently able to expectorate and cough;
  - the patient appears psychologically stable enough to permit adequate cooperation;
  - laryngeal inspection reveals no organically relevant stenosis.
1. Extubation is preceded by administration of an antiphlogistic drug after long-term ventilation.
2. After 20–30 min the pharynx must be cleared by suction, then 6 L/min O_2 given, plus several compressions of a ventilatory bag timed to coincide with the patient's own breathing rhythm. The tube must be withdrawn smoothly and without interruption.
3. 1–3 L/min O_2 should be given via nasal prongs after each extubation.
4. Attentive subsequent care, reassurance of the patient, and assistance in expectoration are necessary.

Extracorporeal Membrane Oxygenation (ECMO)

Principle

- Extracorporeal membrane oxygenation (ECMO) denotes a procedure in which blood is transported past an artificial oxygenator to gain time for restitution of disturbed pulmonary function.
- ECMO is not (or not yet) a routine method, and is reserved as a last-resort procedure in specialized centers.

Indications

- Prerequisite for use of ECMO: potential reversibility of the pulmonary disorder
- Grave hypoxemia with cardiac rhythm disorders and incipient coma
- $PaO_2 < 50$ mmHg at F_{IO2} 1.0 for >2 h, despite optimum PEEP ventilation
- $PaO_2 < 50$ mmHg at F_{IO2} 0.6 for >12 h, despite optimum PEEP ventilation
- Very high airway pressure (danger of barotrauma) that fails to improve when the ventilation pattern is changed
- Potential indication: reduction of pulmonary circulation during bypass may facilitate pulmonary healing by providing relief

Equipment – Technique

- Bypass may be done as follows:
  - Arteriovenously, using the heart as a pump. Drawback: limited flow through the oxygenator.
  - Venovenously. Drawback: O_2-laden blood recirculates, and pulmonary circulation is not reduced.
  - Venoarterially (the most widely practiced method). An adequate supply of O_2 to the left ventricle and the coronary arteries must be assured.
- Reduction of F_{IO2} must proceed by increments. Blood gas analysis from the right radial artery provides orienting data on the cerebral blood supply.

Complications

- Hemorrhage
- Infection
- Mechanical failure

- Maintenance of circulation (closed-chest compression) and/or restoration of normal cardiac rhythm (electrical countershock, electrical pacing)
- Maintenance of respiratory function (ventilation)

Indication

Cardiocirculatory arrest (see p. 60)
Remember:
Resuscitation must be initiated no later than 5 min after occurrence of cardiocirculatory arrest, if in any way feasible. Otherwise, irreversible brain damage is likely; in extreme cases, cerebral death.

External Cardiac Compression (Closed-Chest Compression)

Principle

Two basic mechanisms are involved:
- Rhythmic compression of the heart between the sternum and vertebral column
- Rhythmic variation of intrathoracic pressure
In effect, pressure causes ejection of blood from the heart into the vascular system. When pressure is released, blood flows from the atria to refill the ventricles.

Technique

- The patient is placed supine on a hard surface (floor, table, board inserted into the bed).
- For prolonged closed-chest compression: A mechanically driven external cardiac compressor is used.
- *Methods:*
  1. *Manual closed-chest compression:*
     - The rescuer stands or kneels at the victim's side.
     - Rescuer's arms are extended at the elbows.
     - Pressure point is the lower third of the patient's sternum.
     - The rescuer places the heels of his hands, one over the other, on the pressure point.
     - Applying his own body weight, the rescuer exerts vertical pressure to the sternum to move it about 5 cm closer to the vertebral column.
     - Compression is rhythmic, with pressure and release phases of about equal duration.

    – Frequency is about 80–100/min.
    – Efficacy is monitored by palpating the femoral pulse.
    – Ratio to artificial respiration rate 5:1 if 2 rescuers are present, or 15:2 with only 1 rescuer.
2. *Mechanical heart massage:*
    – The patient's trunk is placed on a special table.
    – The piston is placed on the lower third of the patient's sternum.
    – Excursion amplitude and frequency are adjusted as desired.
    – The machine is turned on.
Remember:
Mechanical heart massage also permits artificial respiration at a rate of 5:1.

- *Signs of successful resuscitation:*
  – Palpable major arterial pulses
  – Pink skin hue and rewarming of skin
  – Constriction of pupils
  – Positive pupillary response to light
  – Return of muscle tone
  – Resumption of spontaneous respiration
  – Spontaneous muscle activity
  – Return of consciousness
  – Measurable arterial blood pressure
  – Return of urine output

Complications:
– Fractures of sternum and/or ribs (in about $\frac{1}{3}$ of cases)
– Hematothorax, pneumothorax, hematopericardium
– Splenic or hepatic rupture
– Gastric mucosal laceration
– Hemorrhage and hematomas of the thoracic wall, subepicardially, subendocardially, of the pericardium, mediastinum, subpleurally, of the adventitia of large vessels, the hepatic capsule, diaphragm, or retroperitoneal space
– Bone marrow embolism
– Fat embolism
– Pulmonary edema
Electrotherapy (see pp. 282, 284)

Mouth-to-mouth resuscitation and use of manual resuscitator

Principle

Insufflation of air from the rescuer's lungs (mouth-to-mouth artificial respiration) or from a manual resuscitator bellows

Cardiopulmonary Resuscitation

Indications

- Respiratory standstill in:
  - Cardiocirculatory arrest
  - Airways obstruction
  - Central respiratory paralysis due to trauma or poisoning
  - Peripheral respiratory paralysis due to neuromuscular paralysis or medication
- Severe respiratory failure in:
  - Shock
  - CO poisoning
  - Global respiratory failure

Technique

- *Preparations:*
  Clear the airways by:
  - overextending the head at the neck,
  - pulling the lower jaw forward and opening the mouth,
  - sweeping the mouth and pharynx clear with a finger.
- *Procedure:*
  Mouth-to-nose resuscitation:
  - Rescuer kneels next to patient's head.
  - Rescuer places one hand on the patient's forehead, the other under the chin.
  - The patient's lower jaw is pulled forward and pressed against the upper jaw.
  - Rescuer seals the patient's nose with his mouth.
  - Rescuer insufflates at a rate of 12–15/min, duration 1–1.5 s.

  Mouth-to-mouth resuscitation:
  - Rescuer kneels next to the patient.
  - Rescuer places one hand on patient's forehead, the other under his chin.
  - Patient's lower jaw is pulled forward, leaving the mouth slightly open.
  - Rescuer seals the victim's mouth with his own.
  - Rescuer uses his cheek to close off the victim's nostrils.
  - Rescuer inflates at a rate of 12–15/min, duration of each inflation 1–1.5 s. Exhalation by the patient is passive.

  Mouth-to-tube resuscitation (e.g., Safar-type oropharyngeal tube):
  - Insert the mouthpiece into the patient's mouth.
  - Standing behind the patient's head, the rescuer tilts it backward.
  - With his middle, ring, and little fingers, the rescuer grasps the patient's lower jaw from below and pushes it forward.

- Using an index finger, the rescuer pushes the sealing plate of the tube firmly over the patient's mouth.
- Rescuer's thumb is used to seal the patient's nose.
- Rescuer exhales into the external opening of the tube.
- Frequency and rhythm are the same as in mouth-to-mouth respiration.

Mouth-to-mouth resuscitation:
- Rescuer kneels behind the patient's head.
- Patient's jaw and chin are grasped from below and pushed forward, while the head is bent backward.
- Rescuer presses the mask firmly over the patient's face, and inflates air into the external orifice of the mask.
- Frequency and rhythm are the same as in mouth-to-nose respiration.

Manual resuscitator-to-mask ventilation (valve-equipped manual resuscitator or mask):
- Attach mask to the resuscitator bellows via the valve.
- Rescuer kneels or stands behind the patient's head.
- With the middle, ring, and little fingers of one hand, rescuer grasps the patient's jaw from below, advances it forward, and tilts the head backward.
- The thumb of the same hand grasps the mask cranially, pressing it over the patient's nose and mouth with the aid of the index finger.
- The other hand pumps the manual resuscitator.

Complications

- Inflation of the stomach (usually when the head is not bent backward sufficiently), which leads to vomiting and aspiration of gastric contents.
- Pharyngeal tubes may elicit choking, vomiting, or laryngeal spasms, and cause damage to teeth.

Pericardiocentesis

Indications

- Diagnostic: pericardial effusions of uncertain origin
- Therapeutic: decompression of the heart

Principle

- Introduction of a cannula or catheter into the pericardial cavity and aspiration of a small amount (diagnostic pericardiocentesis) or nearly the entire fluid content (therapeutic pericardiocentesis)

Equipment – Technique

- *Preparation:*
  Monitoring of circulation: ECG, arterial pressure, 1- or 2-dimensional echocardiography; cardiovascular drugs, defibrillator and ventilation apparatus at hand
- *Instruments:*
  Disinfectant, local anesthetics, lancet or pointed scalpel, ECG equipment, cable bearing an alligator clamp, 20-mL hypodermic syringe, 3-way stopcock, short-beveled puncture needle, wound dressing.
- *Technique:*
  - Place patient in semierect, supine position.
  - Puncture site: Disinfect the skin over the angle formed by the xyphoid and left costal arch.
  - Give local anesthesia.
  - Make stab incision.
  - Attach the puncture needle to a unipolar chest lead via the connecting cable bearing the alligator clamp.
  - Connect the hypodermic syringe to the puncture cannula via the 3-way stopcock.
  - Inject the puncture needle and advance it in the direction of the right shoulder while applying constant suction.
  - Constant ECG monitoring: Elevation of the PQ and ST segments indicates myocardial contact. Position of the cannula may also be monitored by 2-dimensional echocardiography.
  - Retract the cannula a few mm.
  - Withdraw the effusion fluid into the syringe, close the 3-way stopcock, and expel the aspirated fluid into a receptacle. Restore passage to the 3-way stopcock syringe.

Alternative procedure:
- Insert a Seldinger wire, soft end first; advance it into the pericardial cavity and withdraw the cannula. Insert an introduction set along the Seldinger wire. Following withdrawal of the Seldinger wire, a pigtail catheter is inserted in its stead. The pigtail catheter is advanced around the left border of the heart into the posterolateral pericardial recess.
- Following completion of withdrawal of effusions: The cannula or pigtail catheter is withdrawn while applying constant suction, a small dressing applied, and heart and lungs auscultated for signs of pneumothorax.
  Or:
- The catheter is left in situ for long-term pericardial drainage. The catheter is closed off and the pericardial cavity evacuated at intervals by suction.

Complications

- Ventricular tachycardia or fibrillation
- Pneumothorax
  Remember:
  Pericardiocentesis is contraindicated during anticoagulation therapy.

Intraaortic Balloon Counterpulsation

Principle

- ECG-controlled rhythmic filling and deflation of a balloon advanced into the aorta via the femoral and thoracic arteries. The diastolic filling elevates arterial pressure, thus improving coronary perfusion. The balloon collapses during systole, reducing the afterload. The result is more complete emptying of the ventricles and augmentation of cardiac output by 10–20%.

Indications

- Therapy-resistant cardiogenic shock
- As a presurgical precaution in severe unstable angina pectoris with evolving myocardial infarction or in ventricular septal defect or rupture of papillary muscle consequent upon infarction
- Postoperatively in patients completely dependent on a heart-lung machine after valvular replacement or aortocoronary bypass surgery

Technique

Two methods: Percutaneous puncture or puncture after surgical exposure of the femoral artery

- Percutaneous puncture:
  - Stab incision
  - Puncture of the femoral artery
  - Introduction of a spiral guidewire
  - Removal of the trocar
  - Insertion of the introduction set along the spiral guidewire
  - Removal of the spiral guidewire and dilator
  - Advancement of the balloon catheter through the introduction set to the thoracic artery just below the departure of the left subclavian artery
- Surgical technique:
  - Exposure of the femoral artery and insertion of a dacron prosthesis
  - Introduction of the balloon catheter and advancement into the thoracic artery just below the origin of the left subclavian artery
  - Attachment of the catheter to the prosthesis by sutures
  - Wound closure by cutaneous sutures

Regardless of which approach is used, it is followed by attachment of the balloon catheter to the pump and adjustment of the balloon pump.

Complications

- Aortic dissection upon introduction of the catheter
- Intraaortic rupture of the balloon
- Thrombosis near the iliofemoral system
- Hemorrhage (e.g., due to diminution of platelet count)
- Severe mechanical hemolysis
- Infection
- Overdependency on the pump (In such cases heart surgery must be contemplated.)

Remember:

Intraaortic balloon counterpulsation is feasible only in large centers with facilities for heart surgery.

Therapy should be tapered off, not terminated abruptly. The prognosis is highly unfavorable if hemodynamic improvement fails to occur within the first 24–48 h.

Electrical Countershock (Cardioversion)

Principle

- Release of a high-energy (up to 400 WS) capacitor charge to the thoracic wall (duration of about 0.01 s).
  Effect: simultaneous depolarization of the entire heart tissue ("synchronization"). Thereafter, the region with the greatest intrinsic automaticity, i.e., the sinoatrial node, assumes the role of pacemaker.
- Except in ventricular fibrillation, the capacitor is timed for release outside of the ventricle's vulnerable phase, so as not to elicit ventricular fibrillation.

Indications

- Ventricular fibrillation (to defibrillate)
- Atrial fibrillation, atrial flutter
- Paroxysmal supraventricular tachycardia
- Ventricular tachycardia
  Remember:
  Electrical countershock is indicated particularly when the above rhythm disorders have lead to complications, e.g., hypotension, myocardial ischemia, or clouding of consciousness, or when they fail to respond to antiarrhythmic drugs.

Technique

- *Preparation:*
  - Supine position of the patient
  - If the patient is conscious, short-term general anesthesia or deep sedation (e.g., with diazepam IV or midazolam IV)
  - Removal of hair from the chest by shaving
- *Instruments:*
  - Cardioverter with attached electrodes
  - Contact paste
  - ECG recorder or monitor
  - Narcotics or sedatives
  - Hypodermic syringes, needles, gauze sponges
- *Procedure:*
  - Place the ECG leads.
  - Plug cardioverter into house current and switch it on.
  - Check the triggering mechanism (not necessary for ventricular fibrillation).

- Load the capacitor. Selection of discharge energy depends on the type of rhythm disorder to be treated:
  a) For atrial flutter, paroxysmal superventricular tachycardia, or ventricular tachycardia, start at 50 WS.
  b) For atrial or ventricular fibrillation, start at 50 WS or 200 WS, respectively.
- Apply a generous coat of contact paste to the entire contact surface of both electrodes.
- Placement of the electrodes:
  a) If 2 ventral electrodes are used, one is applied at the base of the heart, and the other at the apex.
  b) If a ventral and a dorsal electrode are used, the ventral electrode is applied to the left sternal border between the base and the apex of the heart, and the dorsal electrode below the apex of the left scapula.
- Discharge the capacitor.
- Assessment of the ECG:
  a) Successful electrotherapy: Continue treatment medicinally.
  b) Unsuccessful electrotherapy: Repeat, using a higher-energy discharge.

Complications

- Postdefibrillation rhythm disorders: supraventricular extrasystoles, ventricular extrasystoles, ventricular tachycardia, ventricular fibrillation. Predisposing factors: previous intake of digitalis or quinidine; hypokalemia
- Cardiac arrest
- Arterial embolism (following normalization of atrial fibrillation in patients not previously on anticoagulants)
- Cutaneous burns

Principle

- For bradycardia, direct stimulation of the ventricle at an appropriate rate (70–80/min)
- For tachycardia, interruption of the re-entry circuit by one or more electrical impulses

Indications

- Bradycardic rhythm disorders, e.g.:
  - 2nd- or 3rd-degree AV block,
  - Sick-sinus syndrome
  - Bradycardic atrial fibrillation
  - Hypersensitive carotid-sinus syndrome, accompanied by any of the following:
  - Heart rate below 40/min
  - Syncope
  - Heart failure
- Tachycardic rhythm disorders, e.g.:
  - Atrial flutter
  - Paroxysmal supraventricular tachycardia, including WPW tachycardia
  - Ventricular tachycardia that is refractory to medication

Technique

- *Preparations:*
  - For external (transthoracic) pacing: cleansing of the skin with tap water
  - For transesophageal pacing: anesthesia of the oropharynx (optional)
  - For internal (endocardial) pacing: lokal skin disinfection and local anesthesia of skin over a suitable vein.
- *Equipment:*
  - For external (transthoracic) pacing: large adhesive electrodes
  - For transesophageal pacing: multipolar esophageal electrode
  - For internal (endocardiac) pacing: IV introduction set, electrode catheter, local anesthetic, disinfectant, hypodermic syringes, needles, sponges, protective drapes, sterile gloves, and gown.
- *External (transthoracic) pacing:*
  - Apply the adhesive electrodes to the thoracic wall (precordially adjacent to the left sternal border, and below the left shoulder blade adjacent to the spinal column).

- Select the desired impulse rate and determine the stimulus threshold (usually $>40\,mA$), then adjust the impulse amplitude to approximately 10% above that level.
- Stimulus acts on the ventricle, and may be given for all types of bradycardic rhythm disorders. It is less effective for ventricular tachycardia due to rate limitations and impossibility of programmed pacing.
- Advantage: noninvasive, easily performed method; no antiseptic conditions or x-ray controls are required.
- Drawbacks: Thoracic muscles may contract, causing discomfort to the patient; selective atrial pacing is not feasible.

- *Transesophageal pacing:*
  - Insertion of the esophageal electrode (via mouth or nose) into the esophagus (about 35 cm)
  - Recording atrial or ventricular potentials
  - Connection to the current source; bipolar stimulation by the electrodes recording the highest atrial or ventricular potentials. Initial voltage: $>20\,V$
  - Action of stimulus on the left atrium and left ventricle (the latter is not always possible)
  - Advantages: unsterile procedure, no x-ray controls, no contraction of thoracic muscles. Particulary well-suited for atrial pacing in sick-sinus syndrome or supraventricular tachycardiac arrhythmias, e.g., paroxysmal supraventricular tachycardia, WPW tachycardia, or atrial flutter
  - Drawbacks: risk of trauma to the esophagus. Since ventricular pacing not always successful, usefulness in AV conduction disorders limited

- *Internal (endocardial) pacing:*
  - Puncture a vein (a brachial vein, femoral vein, or subclavian vein).
  - Insert the introduction set.
  - Advance the electrode catheter under x-ray control (if unavailable or not feasible, use intracardiac ECG [see p. 38]):
    a) into the right atrium in supraventricular tachycardia;
    b) into the right ventricle in bradyarrhythmia and ventricular tachycardia.
  - Connect the catheter electrode to the pacemaker system.
  - Remove the introduction set. Apply a dressing, and attach the electrode and the pacemaker firmly.
  - In bradyarrhythmias: Stimulate at a constant rate (70–80/min). Stimulus voltage should not exceed $1\,V$, and the current should be no more than $1.5\,mA$. Voltage and current for stimulation should be set at 3–5 times threshold levels. The sensitivity of the triggering system must be adjusted on demand settings.

– In tachyarrhythmias, a programmed pacemaker is best. First, trigger single discharges (exception: atrial flutter requires at least 3 impulses). If tachycardia persists, give 2 more premature impulses. If this fails, 3 or 4 impulses.

If this too fails (e.g., in most cases of atrial flutter): Apply high-rate stimulation.

Complications

- External (transthoracic) pacing: skin irritation, ventricular fibrillation

- Transesophageal pacing: trauma to the esophagus, atrial fibrillation or flutter, ventricular fibrillation

- Internal (endocardial) pacing:
  – Thrombophlebitis if temporary pacing is kept up for a long period
  – In atrial pacing: atrial fibrillation or flutter; perforation of the atrium
  – In ventricular pacing: ventricular fibrillation; perforation of the ventricle
  – Dislocation of the pacing electrode, resulting in intermittent stimulation or none at all; occasionally, knotting of the catheter within the ventricle
  – Elevation of the stimulus threshold with loss of pacing effect if the electrode has been indwelling for several days

Cardiac glycosides

- Mode of action:
  - Enhancement of myocardial contractility
  - Slowing of AV nodal conduction
- Indications:
  - Acute or chronic heart failure
  - Supraventricular tachycardias
- Contraindications:
  - Impaired AV nodal conduction
  - Sick-sinus syndrome
  - Atrial fibrillation or flutter in WPW syndrome
  - Digitalis-induced rhythm disorders
  - Asymmetric septal hypertrophy
- Adverse reactions:
  - GI: loss of appetite, nausea, vomiting, diarrhea
  - Cardiac: ventricular extrasystoles, sinus bradycardia, supraventricular tachycardia, AV nodal conduction disorders.
- Dosage (IV administration):
  a) Loading dosage in a previously untreated patient: 0.8–1.5 mg, followed by:
  b) Approximate daily maintenance dosage:
  - Digoxin   0.375 mg
  - Digitoxin   0.1 mg
  Dosage in patients with atrial fibrillation depends on the ventricular rate.

Dopamine

- Mode of action:
  - Direct adrenergic action: stimulation of both alpha and beta-1-adrenergic receptors (Small doses evoke only slight vasoconstriction, whereas large doses [> 10 µg/kg/min] are followed by marked constriction of peripheral vessels.)
  - Indirect adrenergic action via liberation of norepinephrine
  - Stimulation of dopamine receptors and consequent dilatation of mesenteric and renal vessels (enhanced urinary output)
- Indications:
  - Cardiogenic shock with marked hypotension
  - Other types of shock if basic therapy fails (volume replacement, correction of acidosis, O_2 administration)
  - Maintenance of urinary output in positive-pressure ventilation and in incipient renal failure

- Contraindications:
  - Thyrotoxicosis, pheochromocytoma, glaucoma
  - Asymmetrical septal hypertrophy
  - In cardiogenic shock following septum perforation, sodium nitroprusside to be tried first
- Adverse reactions:
  Elicitation of extrasystoles and/or acceleration of heartrate
- Dosage:
  Solutions for IV infusion containing 50 and 200 mg: 2–10 µg/kg/min as IV drip

Dobutamine

- Mode of action:
  - Stimulation primarily of beta-1-adrenergic receptors, and to a lesser extent of beta-2- and alpha-adrenergic receptors; no effect on dopamine receptors
- Indications:
  - Advanced heart failure
  - Cardiogenic shock without severe hypotension
- Contraindications:
  - In cardiogenic shock with marked hypotension, dobutamine to be given only in combination with dopamine
  - Asymmetrical septal hypertrophy
  - In cardiogenic shock due to septal perforation, sodium nitroprusside to be tried first
- Adverse reactions:
  - Acceleration of heartrate, extrasystolic beats
- Dosage:
  - 2.5–10 µg/kg/min as IV infusion

Norepinephrine

- Mode of action:
  - Stimulation of alpha-adrenergic receptors and, to a lesser extent, of beta-1-adrenergic receptors; most important: enhancement of peripheral resistance and elevation of blood pressure; improvement of coronary and cerebral circulation
- Drawbacks:
  - Constriction of renal vessels, with consequent reduction of renal circulation and decreased urinary output
  - Augmentation of cardiac O_2 requirements owing to elevated peripheral resistance
- Indication:
  - Marked hypotension in shock

- Contraindications:
  - Ventricular arrhythmias, extrasystolic beats
- Dosage:
  10–100 µg/min as IV infusion
  Remember:
  Dosage and duration should be kept as low as possible.
  Combination with other catecholamines (dopamine, dobutamine) is advisable.

Amrinone

- Mode of action:
  - Enhancement of contractility (Exact mechanism has not been fully elucidated.)
  - Reduction of preload and afterload
- Indication:
  - Myocardial failure that fails to respond to cardiac glycosides, diuretics, and vasodilators
- Contraindications:
  - Obstructive valvular disease
  - Asymmetrical septal hypertrophy with obstruction
  - Marked hypovolemia
  - Ventricular tachycardia and supraventricular tachycardia with rapid ventricular contraction rate
  - Thrombocytopenia
  - Severe impairment of renal function (creatinine in excess of 4 mg/dL)
  - Pregnancy and lactation
- Adverse reactions:
  - Enhancement of the enzymes GOT, AP (alkaline Phosphatase), and LDH (lactate dehydrogenase).
  - Cholestasis.
  - Thrombocytopenia
  - Supraventricular and ventricular tachycardias
- Dosage:
  Bolus injection of 0.5–0.75 mg/kg over 2–3 min; may be repeated after 10–15 min
  Maintenance dose: 5–10 µg/kg/min; maximum daily dosage: 10 mg/kg
  Remember:
  - Individualization of dosage
  - Duration of therapy: maximum of 14 days
  - Dilution only with normal saline (incompatible with glucose)
  - Application via injection into a large vein or via a central IV line

Vasodilating Drugs

Sodium Nitroprusside

- Mode of action:
  - Reduction of cardiac preload by dilation of capacitance vessels
  - Reduction of cardiac afterload by diminution of peripheral resistance due to direct relaxation of arterioles
- Indications:
  - Critical hypertension
  - Reduction of afterload in cardiac pump failure
- Contraindications:
  - Failure of cardiac pumping with hypotension
- Adverse effects:
  - Marked hypotension
  - Cyanide toxicity if large amounts (in excess of 1000 μg/min) are given (caution is also advised with dosages of 500–1000 μg/min)
  - Thiocynate intoxication if administration is prolonged (>2 days)
- Dosage: 20–900 μg/min (maximum)

Nitrates

- Mode of action:
  - Reduction of preload by dilation of capacitance vessels
  - Less marked: reduction of afterload by dilation of arterioles
- Indication:
  Failure of pumping function involving marked elevation of filling pressure
- Contraindication:
  Pumping failure with filling pressures below 20 mmHg (nitrates may cause a further decrease in cardiac output)
- Adverse reactions:
  Headache, hypotension
- Dosage:
  - Nitroglycerin: 10–100 μg/min as IV infusion

Table **23** Vaughan-Williams classification of antiarrhythmic drugs

Class	Mode of action	Clinically relevant target tissue	Drugs for emergencies
I A	Sodium antagonism	Atrium Ventricle	Procainamide
I B	Sodium antagonism	Ventricle	Lidocaine Mexiletine
II	Beta-adrenergic blockade	AV node	see p. 292
III	Potassium antagonism	Atrium AV node Ventricle	Amiodarone*
IV	Calcium antagonism	AV node	Verapamil

* Only in exceptional cases suitable as emergence medication

Lidocaine

- Mode of action:
  - Suppression of ventricular ectopy
  - Decreased automaticity of ventricular pacemakers (No effect on normal AV conduction)
- Indications:
  - Ventricular premature beats
  - Ventricular tachycardia
- Contraindications:
  3rd degree AV nodal block with wide ventricular complexes
- Adverse reactions:
  Usually CNS-related: confusion, fatigue, lethargy, paresthesias, (rarely) seizures
- Dosage:
  Lidocaine in or 2% solution: in ventricular tachycardia 50–100 mg (about 1 mg/kg BW) as IV bolus injection; may be repeated after 5–10 min
  To treat ventricular premature beats and prevent ventricular tachycardia: 100 mg as bolus, repeated after 10 min, followed by infusion: 1–4 mg/min

Procainamide

- Mode of action:
  - Deceleration of conduction rate in cardiac working muscle and in the His-Purkinje system
  - Suppression of automaticity in ectopic pacemakers
- Indications:
  - Ventricular tachycardia
  - WPW tachycardia
  - Atrial fibrillation or flutter in WPW syndrome
- Contraindications:
  - 2nd- or 3rd-degree AV block
  - Caution must be exercised in the presence of bundle-branch block and in heart failure.
- Adverse reactions:
  QRS widening, hypotension, negative inotropic effect
- Dosage: 50–100 mg/min injection with ECG monitoring; stop when QRS duration exceeds initial length by 20%. Load with 10–20 mg/kg slowly over 30–45 min.

Beta-Receptor Blockers

- Mode of action: competitive blockade of beta-adrenergic receptors, resulting in diminished contractility, sinus bradycardia, and AV nodal conduction rate
- Indication: supraventricular tachycardia with rapid ventricular contraction rate
- Contraindications:
  - Disorders of AV nodal conduction; sick-sinus syndrome
  - Myocardial failure in nondigitalized patients
  - Obstructive bronchial disease
  - Systolic blood pressure < 100 mmHg
- Adverse reactions:
  - Slowing of heart rate
  - Myocardial failure
  - Hypotension
  - Bronchial constriction
- Dosage for IV administration:
  - Propranolol: Inject 1 mg/min, maximum initial dose 5–10 mg. Usually given in divided doses of 1–3 mg

Verapamil

- Mode of action:
  Inhibition of calcium influx into myocardial cells, resulting in suppression of sinoatrial nodal automatism and slowed AV nodal conduction
- Indications:
  – Paroxysmal supraventricular tachycardia
  – WPW tachycardia
  – Atrial fibrillation and flutter with high ventricular contraction rate
  – Atrial tachycardia with high ventricular contraction rate
- Contraindications:
  – Supraventricular tachycardia with normal or slowed ventricular contraction rate
  – Myocardial failure
  – Sick-sinus syndrome
  – Arterial hypotension
  – Pretreatment with beta-adrenergic blocking agents
- Adverse reactions:
  Sinus bradycardia, 1st–3rd degree AV block (in extreme cases, asystole), hypotension, myocardial failure
- Dosage:
  Initial dose 5 mg slowly IV; may be repeated after 5–10 min. Maximum daily dose 100 mg

Atropine

- Mode of action: Owing to anticholinergic action, the sinoatrial nodal rate and AV nodal conduction are accelerated.
- Indications:
  - Sinus bradycardia with or without SA block
  - Type-I, 2nd-degree AV nodal block (Wenckebach)
  - 3rd-degree AV nodal block with slender ventricular complexes
  - Atrial fibrillation with low ventricular contraction rate (<50/min)
- Contraindications: glaucoma, prostatic hypertrophy with urinary retention
- Adverse reactions: dryness of the mouth, impaired accommodation, tachycardia
- Dosage: initial dose 0.5–1 mg atropine sulfate

Principle

- Uncritical use of antibiotics and chemotherapeutic drugs has led to the dangerous development of resistant strains. The consequences are particularly deleterious in ICUs. An understanding of resistance and how it develops thus appears relevant.
  Types of resistance:
  – Natural resistance (e.g., of *Pseudomonas* to penicillin)
  – Resistance by mutation prior to initiation of therapy
  – Resistance during therapy following contact with an antibiotic and selection of resistant strains
  – Transmission of resistance from one bacterial strain to another (episomal transmission)
  – Uni- or bilateral cross resistance (particularly relevant in selection of a drug for therapy)

- If therapy with a given antibiotic is ineffective owing to bilateral cross resistance, it makes no sense to administer another antibiotic that is closely related to the first one. When selecting an antibiotic, it is wise to have an alternative drug in reserve in the event that unilateral cross resistance develops.

- In ICUs it is important to keep in mind that otherwise innocuous microorganisms must be regarded as potential pathogens in gravely ill patients, who are highly susceptible to infections and whose immunity is compromised.

Indications

- Antibiotic treatment is indicated when clinical signs of infection are present and bacteriological findings are positive (always considering the patient's overall situation). The only exceptions from this basic rule are:

- Life-threatening conditions, e.g., sepsis, meningitis, or craniocerebral abscesses, in which too much time would be lost waiting for bacteriologic reports. Selection of an appropriate antibiotic is based on the clinical picture and the most likely type of microorganism.
  Remember:
  Even in such cases, samples for microbial culturing and assessment of resistance must be taken *prior* to initiation of therapy.

- In itself, admission of a patient to the ICU does not constitute an indication for antimicrobial therapy. The common practice of preventive administration of broad-spectrum antibiotics in this context is ill-advised.

- Specific, well-planned therapy is the method of choice, not preventive administration. The only indication for systemic preventive administration of antibiotics is short-term perioperative use in major surgery. Such prevention should never be prolonged as therapy.

Medication

- A broad selection of antibiotics is on the market, and frequent introduction of new products makes assessment difficult. In choosing an antibiotic, the specific conditions regarding the problematic microorganism and the patient, as well as activity, pharmacokinetics, application, dosage, and side effects of the drug must be carefully considered. This implies that the antibiotic should be chosen on the basis of its specific action, and also that its spectrum should not be too restricted. In choosing the initial antibiotic, "very broad-spectrum" preparations are just as dangerous for initial treatment as "narrow-spectrum" ones.
  Not every newly-developed antibiotic actually has a new range of specificity. Often the range is merely shifted somewhat.

- Prior to giving an antibiotic, one should review and answer the following questions before making a decision:
  - What is its range of specificity?
  - What is the mode of action?
  - Is there likelihood of cross-reaction?
  - For which organs is it potentially toxic (kidneys, liver, bone marrow)?
  - What possibilities exist for combination?

- Always contemplate single-agent therapy first; do not start off with a combined regimen.
  Keep bacteriocide enhancers such as aminoglycosides in reserve. Primary use of combined antibiotics is usually indicated only in the life-threatening complications mentioned above (sepsis, meningitis, intracranial abscess), in which the results of microbial testing cannot be awaited, or samples for testing are too difficult to obtain.

- Table **24** contains a list of the most frequently-used antibiotics; two antibiotics from each group should be available in an ICU at all times. The list may be added to for specific reasons, depending on the types of patients.

- It is prudent to use only a small selection of antibiotics, in order to be able to relate failures to nosocomial factors.

General Rules

- In initial, nonspecific antimicrobial therapy of a seriously ill patient, the decision as to whether to start with a single agent (selected according to the most likely pathogen in the basic condition and the site of infection) or a combined regimen depends on the severity of the patient's condition.

- Once an antibiogram is available, antibiotic treatment should be as specific as possible, and – if feasible – a combined regimen reverted to single-agent therapy.

- Clinically successful therapy should be maintained.

- Failure to achieve clinical improvement is not necessarily due to choice of an inappropriate antibiotic; above all, additional complications, e.g., sequestration of secretions, aspiration, or abscesses, must be ruled out.

- The usefulness of local application of antibiotics to the oropharynx in preventing pneumonia in ventilated patients cannot yet be definitively assessed. However, recent results seem to support this procedure. It is too early to give well-founded recommendations for specific antibiotics.

Dosage

- In establishing the dosage, pharmacokinetics and potential toxicity of the drugs must be evaluated in the light of any impairment of organ function.
  - This applies particularly to impairment of renal function.
  - The sodium content of certain preparations is high enough to be relevant in patients with congestive heart failure.
  - Computation of dosage in renal failure should be based on creatinine clearance rather than on serum creatinine concentrations.
  - In patients undergoing dialysis, it is relevant to know whether the antibiotic is dialyzable. A large "priming dose" should be given following dialysis.
  - The administration intervals should be reasonable (e.g., q 8 h).
  - Be aware of incompatible combinations.
  - Adhere to the rules given for duration of administration. Give advance written orders regarding the times.
  - Daily maximum dosages and cumulative doses should be noted. This is facilitated by daily addition and careful recording.

- Duration of treatment should not be too brief; avoid arbitrary changes of medication.

- Discontinuation of antibiotics must follow the indication guidelines: bacteriologic and clinical findings, and the overall situation.

297

Table **24** Antibiotics for intensive care units

Group	Approved name	Proprietary name
I. Broad-spectrum penicillins	Azlocillin	Azlin®
	Mezlocillin	Mezlin®
	Piperacillin	Pipracil®
	Ticarcillin and clavulanic acid	Timentin®
II. "Staphylococcus-specific" antibiotics	Oxacillin	Oxacillin®
	Vancomycin	Vancocin®
III. Carbapenemes	Imipenem-cilastatin sodium	Primaxin®
IV. Streptomyces filtrates		
V. Cephalosporins	Cefuroxime	Zinacef® ⎫
	Cefamandole	Mando® ⎬
	Cefoxitin	Mefoxin® ⎭
	Cefoperazone	Cefobid®
	Cefotaxime	Claforan®
	Ceftriaxone	Rocephin®
VI. Aminoglycosides	Gentamycin	Garamycin®
	Tobramycin	Nebcin®
	Netilmycin	Netromycin®
	Amikacin	Amikin®
VII. Gyrase inhibitors		
VIII. Nitroimidazole	Metronidazole	Flagyl®
Antimycotic agent	Miconazole	Monistat®
Virustatic agent	Acyclovir	Zovirax®

Trimethoprim-Sulfamethoxazole is the first-line drug for infection by the facultative pathogen, Pneumocystis carinii, which is becoming increasingly common.

Special features

Bactericidal effect during growth phase
Good regulation with regard to nephrotoxicity
High sodium content

Additional beta-lactamase inhibitor effect of clavulanic acid

For specific use only

Reserve for enterocolitis due to *Clostridium difficile.* Also S. epidermidus

Very wide-range reserve antibiotic

No parallel allergies or resistance to other known substances. High sodium content

"Second-generation" cephalosporins
Bactericidal effect during growth phase
Renal function must be monitored
Effective against *Staphylococcus*
Broad spectrum
Broad spectrum except for Staphylococcus
Convenient administration due to long-lasting effective concentrations

Potentially nephrotoxic, especially in combined regimens
Enhance bactericidal properties of I, II, III, and V
Less ototoxic and nephrotoxic
"Reserve" antibiotic, suitable for single-agent therapy

IV or oral administration
Good penetration of tissues and bone

Effective against anaerobic pathogens

Systemic treatment of severe systemic fungal infections
Herpes virustatic in herpes encephalitis or severe herpes infection in patients with compromised immunity

---

Principle

- For prevention and therapy with immunoglobulins, various preparations are available with different chemical, biological, and immunological properties. The differences are due to various methods of production. Administration may be IV or IM, depending on details of preparation.
- Objective data on specific effects of immunoglobulins are difficult to obtain, and judgment has been based largely on practical experience. Spontaneous changes of course and the influence of other treatment procedures must be considered in evaluation.

Indications

- Prevention of viral and bacteriotoxic diseases. Generally accepted indications either for standard gamma globulin (SGG) or hyperimmune globulin (HIG) are:
  - Viral hepatitis type A   (SG)
  - Viral hepatitis type B   (HIG)
  - Tetanus   (HIG)
  - Rubella   (HIG)
  - Vaccinia   (HIG)
  - Varicella   (HIG)
  - Measles   (SGG)
- As a supportive measure in combined antitoxic and antibacterial treatment during chemotherapy of fulminant infections with a poor prognosis, even in patients without disorders of immunoglobulin synthesis. This indication still awaits definitive confirmation.
  - Severe septic and bacteriotoxic infections require polyvalent gamma globulin containing a wide range of rapidly acting antibodies in high concentrations, long persistence, good clinical tolerance, and freedom from adverse reactions.
  - Such treatment is costly. The indication must be established carefully and early. In any case, administration of antibiotics or chemotherapeutic agents and removal of the cause if possible must not be neglected.

Medication – Dosage

- Aside from the above-mentioned immunoglobulin preparations for specific prevention, a broad range of products especially for the indication "supportive therapy" is available.
  - There is no ideal preparation, despite spectacular success in individual cases. Specific recommendations therefore cannot be given.
  - The choice depends on identification of the immune defects, and may be specific (e.g., in herpes), or based on the antibody spectrum of the preparation and the epidemiologic situation.
  - A critical factor in success of treatment is administration of immunoglobulins in sufficiently large amounts.
  - A single or underdosed administration for economic reasons undermines the efficacy.

Principle

- Critically ill ICU patients are always liable to develop thromboses and consumption coagulopathy with microscopic clotting. Therapy and prevention of thromboembolic complications is feasible with heparin.
  Heparin is effective only in the presence of antithrombin III (AT III); the two form an AT III-heparin complex that neutralizes the effects of thrombin.
- Heparin may be administered in two ways:
  - In amounts appropriate for preventing activation of the coagulation system (*preventive* heparinization), dosed low enough so that PTT and TT remain within normal limits.
  - In amounts large enough to produce detectable anticoagulation (i.e., lengthening of PTT and TT) (*therapeutic* heparinization).

Indications

- *Preventive* heparinization:
  a) Appropriate for every critically ill patient in the ICU, as well as postoperatively and prior to surgery, provided there is *no* overt bleeding or coagulation disorder to contraindicate it
  b) Several important disorders and conditions worth mentioning in particular:
    - Any potential elicitors of disseminated intravascular coagulation, especially conditions involving shock
    - Advanced age
    - Overweight or emaciation
    - Dehydration
    - Varicoses
    - Heart failure
    - Paralysis or palsy
    - Thromboembolic disorders in the case history
    - Pneumonia
    Clearly abbreviated PTT signalizes an enhanced risk of thrombosis.
- *Therapeutic* heparinization:
  Appropriate in all thromboembolic disorders in which there are no contraindications (active bleeding or risk thereof)

Medication – Technique – Dosage

- There are many commercially available preparations derived from biological material which may be given in standardized USP units and are practically nontoxic.

- Low molecular weight heparin has recently become available. Dosage is not yet standardized, and monitoring involves more specific clotting analysis than global tests.

- *Preventive* heparin dosage: 200–500 USP units/h continuously via infusion pump IV, or 5000 IU s.c., b.i.d.

- *Therapeutic* heparin dosage:
  - Bolus of 1000–5000 USP units IV
  - 500–1500 USP units/h IV continuously via infusion pump
  - Laboratory parameters for monitoring efficacy to be checked at desired intervals (at least q 12 h in therapeutic, and q 24 h in preventive administration):
    a) TT is prolonged to 1.5–3 times normal duration, but should not exceed 150 s.
    b) PTT should be above the normal range.
    c) Quick's test should be diminished, but is markedly lower if heparin is overdosed.

- Additional laboratory tests that provide important information:
  - Platelet count (Heparin-induced thrombocytopenia may occur in some cases.)
  - Plasma clotting factors for differentiation of possible clotting disorders
  - Reptilase time for recognition of fibrinolysis (It is influenced *only* by fibrin[ogen] split products, and not by heparin.)
  - Thromboelastogram if disorders of platelet function (thrombopathies) are suspected
  - Heparin concentration when therapeutic doses are given: 0.3–0.8 USP units heparin/mL plasma
  - AT III: Normal level 14–20 mg/dL (Reduction even to 60–70% of the norm (below about 10 mg/dL) may interfere with therapy.)

- Many critically ill patients have a deficiency of AT III that augments the risk of thrombosis.
  - If heparin given in the dosage range of 2000 IU/h fails to prolong PTT and TT, a deficiency of AT III may be involved.
  - Replacement may be accomplished with "fresh-frozen" plasma given q 6–8 h, or concentrated AT III in an initial dose of 1000–2000 IU, followed by 500 IU q 4–6 h thereafter (1 IU is the activity contained in 1 mL fresh plasma).

Complications

- Most frequent complication: hemorrhage due to overdosing or failure to consider the enhanced tendency to bleed when renal function is impaired
- Signs of intolerance (rare)
- Diffuse alopecia (rare)
- Thrombocytopenia (usually not sufficient to force discontinuation of therapy)
- Osteoporosis (occurs in rare cases following long-term treatment)

Subsequent Treatment – Follow-up

- Preventive treatment should be maintained as long as there is a high risk of thrombosis.
- Therapeutic treatment usually lasts for about one week, followed by transition to oral anticoagulants.
  - The transition proceeds in an overlapping fashion with heparin therapy. Heparin may be discontinued when Quick's test drops to <30%.
  - Appropriate physiotherapy cannot be replaced by anticoagulants.

Principle

The term "thrombolysis" refers to enzymatic dissolution of an embolus or thrombus containing fibrin. Degradation of fibrin occurs by proteolytic cleavage of the fibrin molecule by plasmin, the inactive precursor of which is plasminogen. Activation of plasminogen, and thus of the fibrinolytic system, is the principle underlying therapeutic fibrinolysis. Activation may proceed *directly* via transformation of plasminogen to plasmin (endogenous activation, urokinase) or *indirectly* via an activator complex (streptokinase-plasminogen activator complex).

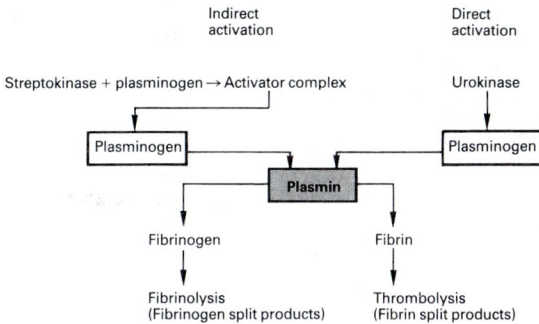

The desired effect is dissolution of fibrin by plasmin within the thrombus. Simultaneous cleavage of fibrinogen (and other plasma coagulation factors) in the bloodstream due to plasminemia contributes to anticoagulation, but also enhances the risk of bleeding.

Streptokinase causes conversion of plasminogen into either plasminogen activator or plasmin. This dual function is responsible for the differing reactive events at various concentrations of streptokinase:

Small amounts of streptokinase → small amounts of activator = marked plasminemia.

Large amounts of streptokinase → large amounts of activator = low plasminemia.

Urokinase follows a dose-response curve.

Indications

- Thrombotic occlusion:
  - Deep venous thrombosis of an iliac or femoral vein that affects the thigh. Lysis is not required if the thrombus extends only to the popliteal vein.
    In thrombotic occlusion limited to an iliac vein, surgical intervention is the first-line procedure.
  - Thrombotic occlusion of a subclavian or axillary vein, depending on the severity of clinical symptoms and on the patient's occupation. Catheter-induced subclavian-axillary venous thrombosis accompanied by marked inflammation is likely to resolve spontaneously following removal of the catheter, so that immediate lysis is not appropriate; bland thrombotic occlusion following long indwelling of the catheter in situ resolves less readily.
  - Fresh occlusions of either renal arteries or veins
  - Occlusions of central retinal artery or vein, but with reservations due to limited experience and lack of clearly defined indications
  - Thrombotic occlusion of extremity arteries not accessible to surgery
  - Fresh coronary artery occlusion
- Embolic occlusion:
  - Pulmonary artery embolism with proximal blockage and acute, fulminant clinical course (acute right heart strain, hypoxemia, reduced peripheral blood flow). Peripherally located pulmonary emboli should be lysed only in exceptional cases.
  - Embolic occlusion of extremity arteries not accessible to surgery
- General considerations in establishing indication:
  1. Age limitation: about 65 years, depending on general condition and on the underlying nonthrombotic disorder
     Exception: acute arterial occlusion with no possibility of surgical intervention
  2. Time of lysis:
     - As early as possible
     - Prospects of success good to excellent if thrombolysis performed within 3 days, particularly in deep femoral and iliac vessels
     - Moderate to poor success likely between the 4th and 12th days, but improves somewhat again in the 3rd–4th weeks; only minimum success expected thereafter
     - Pulmonary embolism: immediately after surgical intervention has been ruled out
     - Coronary artery occlusion: within 4 h of the acute event

Contraindications

Absolute:
– Fresh surgical wounds or trauma (i.e., within the past 7–14 days)
– Translumbar aortography (within the past 4 weeks)
– Arterial puncture and IM injections (within the past 7 days)
– Systemic hemorrhagic disorders (The effects of heparin and oral anticoagulants must have subsided before lysis is begun.)
– Systemic vascular damage, particularly when established. Hypertension in excess of 200/110 mmHg; 2nd degree fundal alterations or worse
– History of cerebrovascular embolism or suspicious present evidence thereof
– Absolute arrhytmia with atrial fibrillation
– Florid endocarditis
– Pregnancy up to the 14th week
– Bleeding hemorrhoids
– Active pulmonary tuberculosis
– Acute pancreatitis
– Cardiopulmonary resuscitation

● *Relative:*
– Old age, poor general condition
– History of hypertension
– Diabetes mellitus
– Puerperium, menstruation, pregnancy beyond the 14th week
– History of ulcers
– Hepatic and/or renal failure
– Severe pneumonia
– Streptococcus infection or streptokinase therapy within in past 3 months (does not apply to urokinase)
– Urolithiasis
– Internal jugular or subclavian venipuncture

Preparation

Prerequisites for thrombolysis:
- Clinical:
  - Thorough physical examination, including neurologic status
  - Phlebographic or scintigraphic evidence of vascular occlusion
  - Clear evidence of myocardial infarction
- Laboratory:
  - Quick's test, PTT, TT, fibrinogen,
    reptilase time, RBC, Hct, Hb, platelet count ⎫
    Urinalysis (sediment)   ⎬ Mandatory
    Blood typing, cross-matched blood in readiness ⎭
  - FSP (fibrinogen split products), plasminogen, ⎫
    plasma clotting factors   ⎪
    Serum transaminases   ⎬ Optional
    BUN   ⎪
    Streptokinase resistance test   ⎪
    (history of streptococcal infection)   ⎭

Medication

- *Streptokinase* – Indirect activation of plasminogen
  Advantage: efficacy and dosage largely proven by many years' experience
  Drawback: difficult to regulate if complications occur; may be antigenic
- *Urokinase* – Direkt activation of plasminogen.
  Advantage: easily regulated; lack of antigenicity
  Drawback: optimum dosage cannot be determined schematically; several times more expensive

Technique – Dosage

Administration of either drug continuously (infusion pump) via a centrally placed, peripherally inserted IV catheter (chest x-ray to verify position of catheter tip); peripheral IV catheter in exceptional cases only

- Procedure for *Streptokinase:*
  Dosage according to a standard protocol with adjusted maintenance dose:
  Initially: 250,000 IU in 5% D/W over 15–30 min
  Thereafter: 100,000 IU in 5% D/W
  Gradually reduce by increments of 20,000 IU if lytic activity in the bloodstream is excessive (assessment of plasma clotting factors) or augmentation of dosage if lytic activity in plasma is deficient (also determined by assessment of plasma clotting factors). Do not

change dosage too hastily (double-check laboratory data, e.g. on blood samples drawn from different sites).
Administer heparin (therapeutic dosage) if there is no response to dosage reduction. Replacement therapy with fresh-frozen plasma or plasminogen and AT III is indicated if lysis has to be continued due to deficient lytic activity.

- Streptokinase dosage in acute coronary occlusion: 0.75–1.5 million IU within 1 h, followed by transition to heparin in therapeutic dosage and oral platelet aggregation inhibitors
- Procedure for *Urokinase:*
  Dosage must be determined individually.
  Initially: 250,000 IU in 5% D/W
  Thereafter: Continue with 100,000 IU, adjusting dosage to meet individual needs (in accordance with reptilase time or thrombin coagulase time). Heparin in therapeutic dosage should be given concurrently, and adjusted in accordance with TT.

  Laboratory monitoring:
  – Coagulation parameters:
    Quick's test, PTT, TT, reptilase time (or thrombin coagulase time) 4–6 h after initiation of therapy, then q 12 h thereafter (PTT should be slightly prolonged to doubled, TT 1½–3 times longer, reptilase time prolonged in comparison to individual baseline value.) } **Mandatory**
  – Blood count, Hct, Hb, urinalysis (sediment) daily to screen for occult bleeding

  – FSP, fibrinogen, plasminogen, AT III, etc. Serum transaminases, electrolytes, BUN q 3 days } **Optional**

  Remember:
  TT is influenced by heparin and split products. Reptilase is influenced by split products, but not by heparin.

- *Duration:*
  5–6 days of therapeutic lysis should be attempted for thrombosis of deep extremity veins. Transition from streptokinase to urokinase + heparin if necessary
  Prolongation of treatment to 14 days if lysis fails in the first 5–6 days (however, chances of success are then below 30%); may be continued longer with urokinase or after transition from streptokinase to urokinase + heparin; 24–48 h lysis for acute, massive pulmonary embolism

Complications

- *Specific complications:*
  - Induction of fever by streptokinase
  - Allergic reaction to streptokinase
- *Nonspecific complications:*
  - Bleeding (usually from sites of injection or wounds)
  - Enhancement of transaminases (streptokinase > urokinase)
  - Confusion, depression
  - Headaches, joint pains
- *Indications for discontinuation of therapy:*
  - Severe, life-threatening hemorrhage due to streptokinase (Microhematuria is an early sign!)
  - *Counteract with:*
    Epsilon-aminocaproic acid 4–5 g IV, followed by 1 g/h for 10 h. Do not discontinue streptokinase before this time. Urokinase should be discontinued immediately.

Superficial bleeding, particularly from injection or puncture sites (compress by sandbag), is *not* an indication for discontinuation of therapy.

Subsequent Therapy

- When therapy is terminated, urokinase or streptokinase should be withdrawn, and heparin (therapeutic dosage) continued (in accordance with TT prolongation).
  - Rapid oral anticoagulation by coumadin (sodium warfarin) monitored by Quick's test (for technical reasons, lower values are obtained during lysis and/or administration of heparin) for 6 months to 1 year after lysis
  - Physiotherapy to restore general physical strength, preferably in a rehabilitation center
  - Monitoring of therapeutic efficacy (including assessment of venous valvular function) by physical examination, determination of venous capacity, Doppler sonography, phlebodynamometry, and phlebography
    Phlebography alone does not provide sufficient evidence of success.

Principle

- Exchange of molecules across a semipermeable filtration membrane for dissolved substances by *diffusion* along a concentration gradient between blood plasma and dialysis fluid. If osmotic pressure of the dialysis fluid exceeds that of the blood, water will be withdrawn from the organism. The same is true when hydrostatic pressure within the blood compartment is greater than that of the dialysis fluid *(ultrafiltration)*.

Clearance by hemodialysis is inversely proportional to molecular weight.

Indications

- Hemodialysis in *chronic* renal failure does not usually fall into the domain of the ICU; its use is governed by unique principles and experience.

Acute hemodialysis is indicated in:

1. Acute renal failure (ARF) of any origin, especially in life-threatening hyperhydration ("fluid lung") and hyperkalemia. Indications in non-life-threatening or polyuric ARF is based on further clinical and laboratory findings (see p. 125).
   - Before initiating hemodialysis, attempts must be made to restore sufficient circulating volume and oncotic plasma pressure (see p. 127), followed by
   - Trial of stimulation with furosemide (500–1000 mg IV as a short infusion, e.g., 30–60 min drip) or ethacrynic acid (0.5–1 mg/kg BW)
2. Acute respiratory failure due to hyperhydration or acute, massive, therapy-resistant heart failure, i.e., for *rapid* withdrawal of water (see also Hemofiltration)
3. Acute exogenous poisoning by a dialyzable substance, provided renal elimination is superior to other procedures, or forced diuresis is ineffectual due to life-threatening circumstances at the beginning or in the course of intoxication
   - Easily dialyzable substances include dissolved salts and alcohols.

     Important indications for individual substances:
     a) Salicylate concentrations > 500 mg/L in serum
     b) Methanol, if intake exceeds 30 mL
     c) Ethylene glycol: always an indication
     d) Ethanol exceeding 4 W/V and/or with respiratory and circulatory collapse
     e) Isopropyl alcohol, if intake exceeded 19 g/kg BW
     f) Thallium if renal function is impaired

4. In combination with hemoperfusion in severe exogenous poisoning (e.g., by paraquat or organic phosphates) with impaired
   renal function

Contraindications

- There are no absolute contraindications. The risks must be weighed
  carefully in prolonged shock and severe clotting disorders.
  Relative contraindications: underlying or secondary disorders car-
  rying an unfavorable prognosis

Preparations

- Verify the indication (exclude postrenal obstruction).
- Obtain informed consent from the patient and/or relatives.
- Provide for balancing and monitoring.
- Position the patient comfortably (supine position). Assure avail-
  ability of a bed scale.
- Plain chest x-ray
- Laboratory:
  Blood count, platelets, Hb, Hct; blood sugar, serum Na^+, K^+,
  Ca^{++}, creatinine, urea; blood gases, cross-matching of blood
- Give written orders for dialysis, specifying amount and type of
  dialysate, heparin-protamine dosage, parameters to be monitored,
  times, and intended duration of hemodialysis, plus projected loss of
  weight.

Technique – Dosage

- Sterile conditions must be provided for establishment of IV access
  route with catheter; a large catheter using Seldinger's technique is
  best.
  1. Insertion of a single needle is possible via:
     - Internal jugular vein
     - Subclavian vein
     - Femoral vein
  2. Two IV lines in case the single-needle access is not feasible: see
     Hemoperfusion, p. 325
  3. Scribner shunt: now used only as an exception, e.g., if frequent
     dialysis appears likely, or placement of a catheter is not feasible
     (loss of time, shunt volume, hazard of bleeding and thrombosis)
- Radiologic verification of catheter position, at least when introduced via subclavian or jugular vein

- Monitoring and procedure of hemodialysis dependent on the indication and the available equipment
- Generally required:
  - Continuous ECG monitoring
  - Blood pressure and pulse taken at 30-min intervals
  - CVP (if feasible) q 2 h
  - Weight control hourly
  - Careful recording of all data!

Heparinization may be local or systemic. Systemic administration of heparin may be continuous or intermittent, but must be intravenous.

Laboratory monitoring:

At least once during dialysis and at termination of each session:

Blood count (including platelets, Hb, Hct), blood sugar, serum levels of Na^+, K^+, Ca^{++}, BUN, blood gases

Remember:

Nephrotoxic drugs that are not vitally essential should be avoided even when hemodialysis is done.

Dosage of drugs must be adjusted according to their elimination by hemodialysis.

Antibiotics should be given *after* each hemodialysis session in a single dose equivalent to an initial dose for a person with intact renal function.

- Duration and frequency of dialysis:
  - Duration: 4–6 h.
  - Frequency: regardless of accumulation of nitrogenous wastes, daily or every second day

Complications

- Cerebral seizures
- Hard-water syndrome
- Febrile reaction
- Hypoxemia of dialysis:
  - Increase availability of O_2
- Hypotension of dialysis:
  - Plasma expansion, cardiovascular drugs
- Thrombocytopenia (usually mild in acute dialysis)
- Hemorrhage:
  - Reduce heparin dosage.
- Hemolysis

Subsequent Monitoring

- Every hemodialysis requires consistent follow-up in keeping with usual ICU criteria.
- Chest x-ray at termination (especially in water intoxication)
- Laboratory monitoring, to include coagulation, electrolyte status, and BUN, a few hours after hemodialysis is completed, as well as just prior to the next hemodialysis session
- The hemodialysis treatment series may be terminated when:
  - Assays indicate that exogenous poisons have been eliminated, and/or clinical findings show that the indication for hemodialysis no longer applies.
  - A previously anuric patient develops polyuria (urinary output > 1000 mL/24 h) and laboratory controls show BUN to be constant or to fall steadily.
- Attempts to enhance renal output by furosemide should be avoided during the hemodialysis series to prevent further tubular damage. If required at all, furosemide should not be given until the series has been completed.
- Careful balancing during the polyuric phase prevents prerenal kidney failure and relapses.

Principle

- Hemofiltration is a procedure for removal of toxic substances from the blood. The driving force for exchange of particles across a filtration membrane is the transmembranous pressure. Transmembranous pressure and molecular separating properties of the membrane determine the type and amount of substances eliminated, regardless of their concentrations. Molecules with a mass of 300–30,000 daltons can be eliminated by hemofiltration. The ultrafiltrate is disposed of and must be artificially replaced.

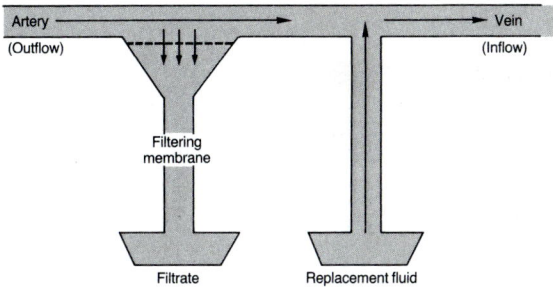

Indication

- Efficacy for elimination of many substances still awaits confirmation by clinical testing.
- Hemofiltration is permissible in:
  - Impairment of renal function and/or conditions involving therapy-resistant water intoxication (acute respiratory failure with hyperhydration, acute massive therapy-resistant heart failure)
  - Intoxication with poisons having a molecular weight of more than 300 daltons, or substances that are filtered by the kidneys, but then reabsorbed
  - Disorders in which separation of plasma and cells is of therapeutic value (see Plasmapheresis, p. 324)

Hemofiltration

Preparation

- Have replacement fluids, albumin, and fresh-frozen plasma at hand for immediate use.
- Provide for monitoring and input-output balancing.
- Laboratory analysis:
  - Hematology with platelet count, Hb, Hct; electrolytes, toxic end products of nitrogen metabolism; electrophoresis; cross-matched blood
  - If feasible:
    Quantitative assessment of poisons in case of intoxication
  - Quantitation of immunoglobulins or immune complexes in auto-immune disorders

Equipment – Technique

Various types of equipment:
- Hemofiltration apparatus with volumetric balancing and replacement of lost fluid
  Routes of access, monitoring, and systemic heparinization as for hemodialysis (see p. 312)
- Modified dialysis apparatus with thermostatic preheating of replacement fluid for extracorporeal dialysis circulation and an additional blood pump for replacement fluid. On the filtrate side, suction is created by a water-driven vacuum pump.
  Routes of access, monitoring, and systemic heparinization as for hemodialysis (see p. 313)
- Dialysis machine plus monitoring and peristaltic pump without dialysis fluid, but with interposition of a suitable hemofilter and catch receptacle, and infusion of albumin and fresh-frozen plasma at the venous limb
- Unmonitored hemofiltration via an artery, with outflow into a vein and constant heparinization. Transmembranous pressure is equivalent to arterial blood pressure, and hydrostatic suction is exerted by the filtrate-containing compartment (so-called arteriovenous hemofiltration).
  Suitable for nonspecialized intensive care units
- Duration of individual treatment and treatment series depends on clinical findings and objective assessment of elimination of substances.

Complications

- Altogether less frequent than in hemoperfusion and hemodialysis, which is a major advantage over the latter procedures.
  – Air embolism
  – Membrane rupture
  – Hyper- and hypovolemia (problem of input-output balancing)
  – Loss of albumen (must be replaced!)
  – Loss of immunoglobulins (must be replaced!)
  – Hypertension
  – Chills and fever
  – Hemorrhage

Subsequent Treatment and Follow-up

- No specific subsequent treatment is required.
- Follow-up examinations, especially of laboratory parameters (as in Preparation) are essential.
- In prolonged treatment, loss of proteins (albumin, globulins) must be given careful attention and replaced if necessary. (Risk of infection is increased due to loss of antibodies.)
- Hepatic laboratory parameters must be monitored, due to possibility of transmission of infections (hepatitis) via fresh-frozen plasma.

Principle

- Hemoperfusion is an extracorporeal detoxification procedure in which grains of active charcoal or ion-exchange resins are perfused by blood. In the process, gases and dissolved substances are adsorbed to the surface of the solids.

Indications

- A distinction should be made between proven and potential indications.
  1. *Proven indications:*
     Severe, acute peroral poisoning with potentially lethal blood levels of substances having low protein affinity, if the response to other procedures is poor or not likely to provide alleviation
     a) *Absolute indications:* paraquat poisoning
     b) *Indications dependent on severity:*
     – Clinical neurologic symptoms of severe poisoning (e.g., Reed IV)
     – EEG (e.g., burst suppression)
     – Critical (i.e., potentially lethal) blood levels (see Table **25**)
     The indication for hemoperfusion is given when *two* of these three criteria are fulfilled.
  Remember:
  Hemoperfusion is no substitute for primary detoxification or basic intensive care.
  Keeping the law of proportionality in mind, never rely on one single criterion (e.g., burst suppression EEG) to justify hemoperfusion.
  2. *Potential indications:*
     Hepatic coma from liver atrophy in:
     – Fulminant hepatitis
     – Toxic, particularly in mushroom poisoning by *Amanita phalloides*

Table **25**   Critical blood levels of some important poisons

Demeton	3 mg/L	Diphenhydramine	10 mg/L
Parathion	0.2 mg/L	Glutethimide	20 mg/L
Dimethoate	1 mg/L	Quinine	10 mg/L
Bromcarbamide	40 mg/L	Digitoxin	80 mg/L
Phenobarbital	100 mg/L	Acetaminophen	200 μg/L
Other barbiturates	50 mg/L	Salicylates	300 μ/L

Preparation

- Stabilize overall condition (cardiocirculatory, respiratory, etc.) as well as possible.
- Laboratory:
  - Hematology (*including* platelet count, Hb, Hct)
  - Clotting status (Quick's test, PTT, TT).
  - Blood typing and crossmatching of 4–6 units of whole blood
  - Serum electrolytes.
  - Toxic end-products of nitrogen metabolism (creatine, urea, uric acid)
  - Blood gases
  - Serum lactic acid
- Supine positioning of the patient (if required, sedation or constraints)

Instruments – Equipment

- Activated charcoal cartridge
- Ion-exchange resin cartridge
- Cartridge containing a mixture of activated charocoal and ion-exchange resins
- Selection of the most suitable cartridge for elimination of a particular poison should depend on most recent information. However, this should not lead to postponement of initiation of hemoperfusion, the type of cartridge being only one aspect of treatment.
- Peristaltic pump or special hemoperfusion apparatus with flow control and pressure manometer
  Optical and/or acoustic alarm capability
  Airtrap
  Arteriovenous tubular system with bubble trap and microfilter

Technique – Dosage

- Puncture of vessels using Seldinger's technique and a large-bore catheter inserted under sterile conditions via:
  - Internal jugular vein or subclavian vein by single-needle method
  - Femoral vessels: veno-venous or arterio-venous (both possible)
  - Femoral vessel/subclavian vein
  - Femoral vessel/jugular vein
  - Subclavian vessel/jugular vein
  Remember:
  Avoid bilateral puncture of subclavian vessels.

319

Permissible:
- Bilateral puncture of jugular veins
- Return of blood via a large-bore *peripheral* catheter

Catheter position must be verified by x-ray.

- Flush tubal system of the cartridge with 1000 ml physiologic saline and 2000 IU heparin

- Tubal system of the cartridge to be filled with 5% human albumin and 2000 IU heparin (superior to saline, especially in presence of blood pressure problems)

- Initially, slow IV injection of 2000 IU heparin dissolved in 10 mL isotonic (0.9%) saline

- Prior to starting, 100 mg prednisolone slowly IV

- Local heparinization:
  - Continuous IV infusion of heparin into the tubal system proximally to the cartridge
  - Continuous IV infusion of protamine into the tubal system downstream from the cartridge

Dosage and rate of infusion must be calculated to leave 500 IU heparin/h unbuffered in circulation (or less if renal function is impaired).

- Start slowly, increasing flow rate until an optimum effect is achieved.

- Monitoring:
  a) Clinical:
  - Blood pressure and pulse: q 30 min
  - Temperature and CVP: hourly
  - Basic intensive care monitoring
  - ECG monitoring

  b) Laboratory:
  - Hematology: CBC (complete blood count), platelet count, Quick's test, PTT, TT, lactic acid (increase possible)
  - Blood gases (P_{aO_2} may drop, predisposing to acidosis.)

  d) Duration of perfusion depends on properties of the cartridge.

Complications

- Hemorrhage:
  - Generalized (particularly in nose and throat)
  - Locally from puncture sites → TT monitoring; increased dosage of protamine if appropriate
  - Clots in tube system of cartridge: reduction of protamine or change of tubal system
  - Allergic reaction → corticosteroids
  - Poor circulation → vasoactive drugs
  - Elevation of pressure or suction in tubal system: flushing of catheter; shunting and change of the catheter if appropriate
  - Thrombocytopenia → discontinuation of therapy at $< 30,000$–$50,000$ → thrombocyte-rich fresh plasma
  - Low P_{aO_2} (usually transitory at start) → increase in rate of O_2 administration
  - Acidosis (usually transitory at start) → correction

Subsequent Treatment – Follow-up

- Leave catheter in situ and perfuse as long as repeated hemoperfusion is planned or likely.
- Monitor coagulation status and hematology (including platelet count). Hemoperfusion is contraindicated when platelet count $< 80,000$–$100,000$.
- Terminate treatment when poison is no longer found in blood or concentrations are minimal. Relate to overall situation.
  Remember:
  Since many substances (especially organic phosphates) are capable of redistribution from tissues into the bloodstream, readiness for hemoperfusion should be maintained up to 24 h following the last blood analysis. In case of poisoning with paraquat, hemoperfusion must be continued until assays of both blood and urine are negative.

Principle

- Peritoneal dialysis makes use of the fact that the peritoneum is a semipermeable membrane through which selective diffusion and filtration of poisons, water, and electrolytes are possible. Dialysate infused into the peritoneal cavity has intimate contact with the peritoneum, thus permitting effective osmotic exchange, depending on the properties of the lavage fluid.
  There are three types of peritoneal dialysis:
  - IPD (intermittent peritoneal dialysis)
  - CPD (continuous peritoneal dialysis)
  - CAPD (continuous ambulatory peritoneal dialysis)
  The procedure of choice in the ICU is CPD.

Indications

- Basically, the range of indications is the same as that for hemodialysis and hemofiltration.
- The main advantage of CPD is technical simplicity, which permits it to be done in hospitals lacking specialized facilities.
  Other advantages include:
  - Heparinization not generally required
  - Gentle withdrawal of fluid and minimal interference with circulation
  - Minor invasiveness
- Drawbacks are:
  - Lower efficiency
  - Greater protein losses
  - Higher risk of hyperhydration
  - Risk of peritonitis

Preparation

- Shaving of the abdomen
- Instruments for paracentesis and fixation of the catheter at hand
- Appropriate dialysis fluid at hand
- Laboratory workup as for hemodialysis

Equipment

- The simplest apparatus consists of an infusion stand with warm perfusion fluid, a connecting-tube system, and a runoff container.
- Semiautomated apparatus
- Fully automated apparatus

Technique

- Following local anesthesia, a stab incision is made between the upper and middle thirds of a line between umbilicus and symphysis, and a stylet-bearing catheter (aseptic precautions, Tenckhoff catheter) is introduced into the abdominal cavity
- Instillation of the perfusion fluid depends on the apparatus. In any case, the initial portion should be delivered rapidly. 1.5–2 L dialysate are permitted to flow in, then carefully drained following a short period of retention. This procedure should be repeated continuously, with breaks according to technical requirements and patient tolerance.
- A negative input-output balance should be approached gradually.
- Monitoring and adjustment are as for hemodialysis.

Complications

- Occlusion or flow hindrance of the catheter: 1000 IU heparin/2 L dialysate in appropriate cases
- Hyperhydration: problem of input-output balance
- Hypokalemia: problem of laboratory monitoring
- Hypovolemia
- Loss of protein
- Hemorrhage
- Perforation
- Peritonitis

Principle

- The goal of plasmapheresis is elimination of plasma proteins and protein-bound toxic substances.
  Plasma is withdrawn and replaced (plasma exchange). The procedure corresponds to hemofiltration with large-pore filtering membranes (so-called plasma filtration).

Indications

- Many indications, particularly those related to immunology, are considered acceptable, although they have yet to be confirmed.
  The following is a selection of important conditions for which the evidence appears to justify plasmapheresis in critical situations:
  1. Immunologic disorders:
     - Goodpasture's syndrome
     - Myasthenia gravis
     - Inflammatory systemic disorders (e.g., SLE, after all other conservative treatment options have been tried)
  2. Guillain-Barré syndrome
  3. Endogenous poisoning:
     - Thyrotoxicosis
  4. Para- and dysproteinemias
  5. Exogenous poisoning by substances readily bound to protein (see also Hemofiltration)

Preparation

- As for hemofiltration (q.v.).

Equipment – Technique

- *Simplest method:*
  - Withdrawal of blood as for transfusion
  - Centrifugation of blood
  - Reinfusion of blood cells and replacement of protein losses
  1. Advantage: minimum organization required
  2. Drawback: limited efficiency due to quantitative restrictions
  3. One central IV catheter is basically sufficient, but 2 separate IV lines permit immediate correction of volume depletion.

- *Gravitational separation of blood cells:*
  - Intermittent blood flow
    Advantage: only one catheter required (single-needle technique)
    Drawback: more time-consuming; problems of input-output balance
  - Continuous blood flow
    Advantage: gradual separation of plasma; hardly any significant problems of input-output balance
    Drawback: 2 catheters of a double lumen single catheter must be used
- Equipment and plasma replacement follow the same principles as *hemofiltration* with large-pore membrane filters (see p. 316).

Complications

- Volume fluctuations
- Hypothermia
- Electrolyte depletion
- Intolerance
- Hemorrhaging
- Antibody depletion

Rewarming in Hypothermia

Principle

- Elevation of body temperature to counteract or prevent complications of hypothermia (See below.)

Indications

- Active rewarming is appropriate in all cases of severe hypothermia (i.e., rectal temperature <32°C).
- Passive rewarming is usually sufficient in moderate hypothermia.
  Remember:
  In critically ill patients, moderately subnormal temperatures (35–36°C) are preferable to elevated temperatures for metabolic reasons.

Technique

- Passive rewarming by increasing the ambient temperature: wrapping in woolen blankets, elevating ambient temperature to 25–30°C
- Active warming from without by a warm bath (temperature gradually increasing from 35 to 40°C) in young, healthy individuals following overexposure to cold.
  Remember:
  Active and rapid external rewarming may be dangerous to the elderly, and is contraindicated after overdosage of sleeping pills.
  Reasons: hypotensive response and increase of acidosis when the surface of the body is warmed while hypothermia of the body core persists
- Active rewarming of the body core:
  - Infusion of warm fluids (39–40°C).
  - Hemodialysis with overwarmed dialysate
  - Cautious rewarming: increase of body temperature by about 1°C/h

Complications

- Cardiac rhythm disorders, in extreme cases ventricular fibrillation.
- Hypotension due to peripheral vasodilation.
- Augmentation of acidosis.
- Local injury to the skin by inappropriate external application of warmth.

Principle

- Symptomatic measures to reduce body temperature, independent of treatment of the underlying disorder
- Hyperthermia involves accelerated metabolism and hyperkinetic circulatory responses:
  - Increased energy turnover
  - Increased O_2 consumption
  - Hyperventilation with hypocapnia (linear correlation between body temperature and P_{aCO_2})
  - Tachycardia
  - Increased cardiac output
- Hyperthermia is very common in critically ill patients; the causes are many and complex:
  - Elevated temperature as part of the pathophysiology of acute, severe disorders regardless of etiology
  - Fever due to infections and infectious complications
  - Excitation stage of sleeping-pill intoxication
  - Certain poisons, e.g., atropine
  - Thyrotoxicosis
  - Craniocerebral trauma

  Remember:

  a) In ICU patients, fever is not automatically equivalent to infection.

  b) Typical bacterial complications in ICU patients include:
  - Pulmonary infection in intubated patients undergoing ventilation
  - Urinary tract infections in patients with indwelling bladder catheters
  - Wound infections
  - Infected puncture sites of indwelling intravascular lines

  The mere presence of pathogens is not sufficient for diagnosis; one should always attempt to distinguish between contamination and infection.
- Septicemia is rarely the primary occasion for admission to an ICU; it develops 3–4 times more often as a complication during ICU treatment. Septicemia is a central factor in the pathogenesis of multiple organic failure: septic lung, septic shock, acute renal failure due to sepsis, septic coma, GI stress bleeding in sepsis, liver atrophy precipitated by sepsis.

Indications

- Body temperature continuously $>39\,^{\circ}C$

Techniques

- Sedatives and drugs that inhibit the autonomic nervous system to reduce production of heat and the body's counterregulation when heat is withdrawn:
- Withdrawal of heat by cooling (in combination with sedatives)
  - Removal of bedcoverings (= lowering of ambient temperature)
  - Fanning (= cooling by convection)
  - Application of cold compresses to extremities and trunk (= withdrawal of heat by evaporation)
  - Application of icebags or chemical cold packs to large superficial vessels (neck, groin) (= cooling of circulating blood)
- Antipyretic medication to influence central thermoregulation. Repeated administration of antipyretics must be avoided because of their well-known side effects. In individual cases, the dangers posed by hyperthermia must be weighed against possible adverse reactions to such drugs.

Principle

- All ICU patients require specific physiotherapy, which as a rule should be provided by physiotherapists and supplemented by ICU nurses and attendants.
- Physiotherapy consists of:
  1. Passive exercises, including:
     - Full excursion of all joints in sedated or – particularly – relaxed patients undergoing ventilation
     - Vibratory massage (manual or electrovibratory) of the thorax (care of the lungs)
  2. Active exercises, including:
     - Breathing exercises
     - Breathing therapy
     - Active isometric and isotonic tension exercises
     - Mobilization, especially following myocardial infarction

Indications and Procedure

- Indications for passive or active physiotherapy are not based on strict guidelines, but rather oriented to individual requirements.
- Personnel engaged in physiotherapy must be informed daily by the physician regarding the patient's disorder, condition, and exercise tolerance.
- A schedule of treatment times must be drawn up and coordinated with the care schedule.
- Two daily treatments of 15 min each, separated by an adequate interval, are optimal.
- Sedated or relaxed patients on ventilation require passive movement at rgular intervals to prevent joint stiffening with or without calcification of capsule and tendons.
- Lightly sedated patients should participate as early as possible in isometric muscle exercises. This is possible even for patients under fairly heavily sedation if commands are given clearly and repeatedly.
- As the patient regains consciousness, a transition from passive to active physiotherapy should be made. During weaning from the ventilation apparatus to spontaneous respiration, emphasis is placed on breathing exercise and chest therapy.
- Mobilization should be initiated only in patients capable of spontaneous respiration, and proceed gradually to walking exercises.

Physiotherapy

Complications

- May result from inappropriate excursion of extremities with IV lines (briefing!)
- Cardiocirculatory complications
  Prevention:
  Presence of experienced nursing personnel, checks by physicians, monitoring of pulse and blood pressure
- Complications due to vague or inappropriate indications in gravely ill patients with multiple organ failure
  Remember:
  Priorities must be set in the absence of sufficiently qualified personnel.
  Physiotherapy is inappropriate during hemodialysis, hemoperfusion, or hemofiltration sessions.

Follow-up Treatment

- Following physiotherapy appropriate for ICU patients, physiotherapy designed specifically for the particular disease entity should be initiated (e.g., follow-up treatments for thrombosis, myocardial infarction: walking, active muscular training).
  Remember:
  Give specific, well thought-out instructions.
  Do not use physiotherapists merely to assist patients in walking.

Index